Cases for PACES

Stephen Hoole MA, MRCP, DM
Consultant Cardiologist
Papworth Hospital
Cambridge
UK

Andrew Fry MA, MRCP, PHD
Consultant Nephrologist and Acute Physician
Addenbrooke's Hospital
Cambridge
UK

Rachel Davies MA, MRCP, PHD
Consultant Respiratory Physician
Hammersmith Hospital
London
UK

Third Edition

WILEY Blackwell

Registered Office
John Wiley & Sons, Ltd, The Atrium, Southern Gate, Chichester, West Sussex, PO19 8SQ, UK

Editorial Offices
9600 Garsington Road, Oxford, OX4 2DQ, UK
The Atrium, Southern Gate, Chichester, West Sussex, PO19 8SQ, UK
350 Main Street, Malden, MA 02148-5020, USA

For details of our global editorial offices, for customer services and for information about how
to apply for permission to reuse the copyright material in this book please see our website at
www.wiley.com/wiley-blackwell

Library of Congress Cataloging-in-Publication Data

Hoole, Stephen, author.
Cases for PACES / Stephen Hoole, Andrew Fry, Rachel Davies. – Third edition.
    p. ; cm.
  Preceded by Cases for PACES / Stephen Hoole ... [et al.]. 2nd ed. 2010.
  Includes index.
  ISBN 978-1-118-98357-7 (pbk.)
I. Fry, Andrew (Nephrologist), author.   II. Davies, Rachel, active 2015, author.   III. Title.
[DNLM: 1. Physical Examination–Examination Questions.   2. Ethics, Clinical–Examination
Questions.   WB 18.2]
  RC66
  616.07'5–dc23

                                            2014049398

A catalogue record for this book is available from the British Library.

Wiley also publishes its books in a variety of electronic formats. Some content that appears in print may
not be available in electronic books.

Set in 7.5/9.5pt Frutiger by SPi Publisher Services, Pondicherry, India
Printed and bound in Malaysia by Vivar Printing Sdn Bhd

1   2015

Contents

Station 5: Brief Clinical Consultations, 117

Foreword

We are – as always – in a time of flux, with medical careers and the organization of hospitals needing to adjust to meet changing demands. But the fundamental essentials of the practice of clinical medicine have not changed at all. The doctor needs to be able to take a history from a patient, examine them and decide whether investigations and/or treatment are required. They then need to be able to discuss the various options with the patient in an appropriate manner, hopefully reaching a sensible mutual understanding about how best to proceed. The doctor may need to give difficult and distressing information, and must learn how to do it in a way that is clear and does not duck the issues, but also does not increase the pain. And all of these things must be done in a reasonable time frame: the next patient is waiting.

The MRCP PACES examination remains the measure that is most generally respected as indicating that a doctor has developed a fair degree of the knowledge, skills and behaviours that are necessary to do the things detailed above. They are not yet the finished article (beware of anyone, including any consultant, who thinks they are), but they can proceed from core to specialist training. The examination is not easy, with a pass rate of around 40%. Those preparing for it need to immerse themselves in clinical work. There is no substitute for seeing a lot of cases and taking histories and performing examinations, but – and here is where books such as *Cases for PACES* come in – endless repetition of sloppy practice isn't helpful. The physician examining you in the PACES examination is thinking: 'Is this doctor ready to be my SpR now? Can they sort things out in a reasonably efficient and sensible way? Would I get a lot of people wanting to see me because problems had been explained or dealt with poorly?'

What comes over in *Cases for PACES* is a pragmatic and sensible approach that sorts the wood from the trees and cuts pretty rapidly to the chase. I recommend it to you: if you do what it says you will stand a better chance of passing the examination than if you do not.

Dr John Firth
Consultant Physician, Addenbrooke's Hospital, Cambridge
PACES Examiner

Preface

PACES (Practical Assessment of Clinical Examination Skills) was initiated in June 2001 by the Royal College of Physicians as the final stage of the MRCP examination. The initial examination consisted of five stations in a carousel: Station 1, Respiratory and Abdominal (10 minutes each); Station 2, History Taking (20 minutes); Station 3, Cardiology and Neurology (10 minutes each); Station 4, Communication Skills and Ethics (20 minutes) and Station 5, Short Cases (Skin, Locomotor, Eyes and Endocrine; 5 minutes each). The format was refined in October 2009 by restructuring Station 5. This station now has two 10-minute 'Brief Clinical Consultations' that encompass the whole exam and draw on the key skills required to be a competent registrar: the ability to extract a succinct and relevant history, elicit the key physical signs, construct a sensible management plan and communicate this to the patient.

Cases for PACES, 3rd edition, prepares candidates for the current PACES examination. It mimics the examination format and is designed for use in an interactive way. The 3rd edition has a completely revised text that has been informed by recent successful candidate feedback. It now has useful advice for the day of the exam and provides updated information on ethical and medicolegal issues. There is plenty of history-taking advice with new examples and mock questions for candidates to practise themselves. Station 5, the newest and perhaps the most challenging of stations, receives more attention than in previous editions.

Avoid further factual cramming at this stage – you know enough! Go and see medical patients on a busy acute medicine unit or outpatient department. This has always been the best way to prepare for PACES and this book will assist you to do this. We now include mock 'mark sheets', designed to enable groups of candidates to practise 'under examination conditions' at the bedside.

Common cases that regularly appear in the exam, rather than rarities, have been deliberately chosen. We assume candidates will be familiar in examination techniques and the appropriate order in which to elicit the various signs. We provide discussion topics on which a candidate could be expected to comment at the end of the case. Examiners are monitoring specifically for knowledge of the differential diagnosis and organized clinical judgement, while managing the patients' concerns and maintaining patient welfare. The detail is not exhaustive but rather what is reasonably needed to pass. There is additional room to make further notes if you wish.

The aim of this book is to put the information that is frequently tested in the clinical PACES examination in a succinct format that will enable capable candidates to practice and pass with ease on the day.

We wish you the best of luck.

Stephen Hoole
Andrew Fry
Rachel Davies

Acknowledgements

We acknowledge the help of Dr Daniel Hodson in the previous two editions. We thank the doctors who taught us for our own PACES examination, and above all the patients who allow us to refine our examination techniques and teach the next generation of MRCP PACES candidates.

Abbreviations

ABG	Arterial blood gas
ABPA	Allergic bronchopulmonary aspergillosis
ABPM	Ambulatory blood pressure monitoring
ACE	Angiotensin-converting enzyme
ACE-I	Angiotensin-converting enzyme inhibitor
ACTH	Adrenocorticotrophic hormone
ADLs	Activities of daily living
AF	Atrial fibrillation
AFP	Alpha-fetoprotein
AICD	Automated implantable cardiac defibrillator
AIH	Autoimmune hepatitis
ADPKD	Autosomal dominant polycystic kidney disease
ANA	Anti-nuclear antibody
AR	Aortic regurgitation
ARB	Angiotensin receptor blocker
ARVD	Arrhythmogenic right ventricular dysplasia
5-ASA	5-Aminosalicylic acid
ASD	Atrial septal defect
AVR	Aortic valve replacement
BIPAP	Bi-level positive airway pressure
BMI	Body mass index
CABG	Coronary artery bypass graft
CAPD	Continuous ambulatory peritoneal dialysis
CCB	Calcium-channel blocker
CCF	Congestive cardiac failure
CF	Cystic fibrosis
CFA	Cryptogenic fibrosing alveolitis
CFTR	Cystic fibrosis transmembrane conductance regulator
CK	Creatine kinase
CML	Chronic myeloid leukaemia
CMV	Cytomegalovirus
COMT	Catechol-O-methyl transferase
COPD	Chronic obstructive pulmonary disease
CRP	C-reactive protein
CSF	Cerebrospinal fluid
CVA	Cerebrovascular accident
CVID	Common variable immunodeficiency
CXR	Chest X-ray (radiograph)
DBP	Diastolic blood pressure
DIPJ	Distal interphalangeal joint
DM	Diabetes mellitus
DMARDs	Disease-modifying anti-rheumatic drugs
DVLA	Driver and Vehicle Licensing Agency
DVT	Deep vein thrombosis
EBV	Epstein–Barr virus
ECG	Electrocardiogram
eGFR	Estimated glomerular filtration rate
EMG	Electromyogram
ESR	Erythrocyte sedimentation rate
FBC	Full blood count

FEV₁	Forced expiratory volume in 1 second
FTA	Fluorescent treponema antibodies
FVC	Forced vital capacity
GH	Growth hormone
Hb	Haemoglobin
HBV	Hepatitis B virus
HCG	Human chorionic gonadotrophin
HCV	Hepatitis C virus
HGV	Heavy goods vehicle
HLA	Human lymphocyte antigen
HOCM	Hypertrophic obstructive cardiomyopathy
HRT	Hormone replacement therapy
HSMN	Hereditary sensory motor neuropathy
HSV	Herpes simplex virus
IBD	Inflammatory bowel disease
IDDM	Insulin-dependent diabetes mellitus
IGF	Insulin-like growth factor
INR	International normalized ratio
ITP	Immune thrombocytopaenic purpura
IV	Intravenous
JVP	Jugular venous pressure
K_{co}	Transfer coefficient
LAD	Left axis deviation
LDH	Lactate dehydrogenase
LFT	Liver function test
LMWH	Low molecular weight heparin
LQTS	Long QT syndrome
LV	Left ventricle
LVEF	Left ventricular ejection fraction
LVH	Left ventricular hypertrophy
LVOT	Left ventricular outflow tract
mAb	Monoclonal antibody
MAO	Monoamine oxidase
MCPJ	Metacarpophalangeal joint
MI	Myocardial infarction
MND	Motor neurone disease
MPTP	Methyl-phenyl-tetrahydropyridine
MR	Mitral regurgitation
MRI	Magnetic resonance imaging
MTPJ	Metatarsophalangeal joint
MVR	Mitral valve replacement
NIPPV	Non-invasive positive pressure ventilation
NSAIDs	Non-steroidal anti-inflammatory drugs
NSCLC	Non-small cell lung cancer
OA	Osteoarthritis
Pₐ	Partial pressure (arterial)
PBC	Primary biliary cirrhosis
PCT	Primary Care Trust
PE	Pulmonary embolism
PEFR	Peak expiratory flow rate
PEG	Percutaneous endoscopic gastrostomy
PET	Positron emission tomography
PIPJ	Proximal interphalangeal joint
PR	Per rectum

PRL	Prolactin
PSA	Prostate-specific antigen
PSC	Primary sclerosing cholangitis
PSV	Public service vehicle
PTHrP	Parathyroid hormone-related peptide
PUVA	Psoralen ultraviolet A
PVD	Peripheral vascular disease
RA	Rheumatoid arthritis
RAD	Right axis deviation
RBBB	Right bundle branch block
RR	Respiratory rate
RV	Right ventricle
RVH	Right ventricular hypertrophy
Rx	Treatment
SBP	Systolic blood pressure
SCLC	Small cell lung cancer
SIADH	Syndrome of inappropriate anti-diuretic hormone
SLE	Systemic lupus erythematosus
SOA	Swelling of ankles
SSRI	Selective serotonin reuptake inhibitor
SVCO	Superior vena cava obstruction
T_4	Thyroxine
$T°C$	Temperature
TB	Tuberculosis
TIA	Transient ischaemic attack
TIMI	Thrombolysis in myocardial infarction
T_LCO	Carbon monoxide transfer factor
TNM	Tumour nodes metastasis (staging)
TOE	Transoesophageal echo
TPA	Tissue plasminogen activator
TPHA	*Treponema pallidum* haemagglutination assay
TR	Tricuspid regurgitation
TSAT	Transferrin saturation
TSH	Thyroid stimulating hormone
TTE	Transthoracic echo
UC	Ulcerative colitis
U&E	Urea and electrolytes
UFH	Unfractionated heparin
UIP	Usual interstitial pneumonia
UTI	Urinary tract infection
VATS	Video-assisted thorascopy
VEGF	Vascular endothelial growth factor
VSD	Ventricular septal defect
WCC	White cell count

Advice

Preparation

Practice makes perfect; it makes the art of eliciting clinical signs second nature and allows you to concentrate on what the physical signs actually mean. Practice makes you fluent and professional and this will give you confidence under pressure. We strongly encourage you to see as many patients as possible in the weeks leading up to the exam. Practice under exam conditions with your peers, taking it in turns to be the examiner. This is often very instructive and an occasionally amusing way to revise! It also maintains your motivation as you see your performance improve. We also encourage you to seek as much help as possible from senior colleagues; many remember their MRCP exam vividly and are keen to assist you in gaining those four precious letters after your name.

The day before

Check that you have your examination paperwork in order with your examination number as well as knowing where and what time you are needed: you don't want to get lost or be late! Also ensure that you have packed some identification (e.g. a passport) as you will need this to register on the day. Remember to take with you vital equipment with which you are familiar, particularly your stethoscope, although avoid weighing yourself down with cotton wool, pins, otoscope, etc. The necessary equipment will be provided for you on the day. Punctuality is important and reduces stress so we advise that you travel to your exam the day before, unless your exam centre is on your doorstep. Avoid last minute revision and try and relax: you will certainly know enough by now. Spend the evening doing something other than medicine and get an early night!

On the day

Think carefully about your attire: first impressions count with both the examiners and – more importantly – the patients. Broadly speaking, exam dress policy is similar to that required of NHS employees. You should look smart and professional, but above all wear something that is comfortable! Shirts should be open collar (not low cut) and short sleeved to enable bare-below-the-elbow and effective hand sanitation. Remove watches/jewellery (wedding bands are permitted) and dangling necklaces/chains that could be distracting. Facial piercings other than ear studs are not recommended.

Examination

Use the preparatory time before each case wisely. When you enter the station remember to 'HIT' it off with the examiners and patient:

- **H**and sanitization (if available),
- **I**ntroduce yourself to the patient and ask permission to examine them,
- **T**ake a step back once the patient is appropriately uncovered/positioned. As soon as you start touching the patient, focus becomes blinkered and you will miss vital clues to the case.

Remember to HIT it off and your nerves will settle, you'll be underway and the rest will follow fluently if you are well practised.

Rather like a driving test when looking in the rear-view mirror, be sure to convey to your examiner what you are doing. Similarly, your examiner will be expecting to see you do things in a certain order. Stick to this and examiner 'alarm bells' will remain silent. However, if you do forget to do something half way through the examination, or you have to go back to check a physical finding, do so. It's more important to be comprehensive and sure of the clinical findings, than simply being 'slick'.

Spend the last few moments of your examination time working out what is going on, what the diagnosis is and what you are going to say to the examiner. There's still time to check again. Most examinations can be completed by standing up and stating to the examiners a phrase like: 'To complete my examination I would like to check…' and then listing a few things you may have omitted and/or are important to the case.

Presentation

Eye contact and direct, unambiguous presentation of the case conveys confidence and reassures examiners that you are on top of things. Avoid the phrases 'I'm not sure if it is…' and 'I think it is…'. Be definitive and avoid sitting on the fence but *above all be honest*. Don't make up clinical signs to fit a specific diagnosis but do not present clinical signs that are inconsistent with the diagnosis or differential diagnosis.

There are two ways to present the case:

* **state the diagnosis and support this with key positive and negative clinical findings** – if (and only if) you are confident you have nailed the diagnosis!
* **state the relevant positive and negative clinical signs (often easier in the order elicited) and then give the differential diagnosis** that is consistent with them – particularly if you are unsure of the diagnosis.

Where possible, a comment on the disease severity or disease activity should be made. Consider complications of the diagnosis and mention if these are present or not. Know when to stop presenting. Brevity can be an asset. It avoids you making mistakes and digging a hole for yourself! Wait for the examiners to ask a question; do not be preemptive – the examiners may follow up on what you say.

Examiners

Prior to you examining the patient the examiners will have individually 'calibrated the case' to ensure that the clinical signs are present. This maintains the fairness and robustness of the exam and makes sure consistency exists between exam centre marking. There will be two examiners for every carousel station and usually one will lead the discussion with you. Both will have mark sheets and will mark you individually without collaboration. Contrary to popular belief they both want you to pass. They are there because they support the college training and progression of talented physicians of the future.

Mistakes happen

If you do make a mistake and realize it, do not be afraid to correct yourself. To err is human and the examiners may overlook a minor *faux pas* if the rest of the case has gone well. It is not uncommon to think you have failed a case half way round the carousel and that your chances of passing PACES has been dealt a fatal blow. We are often our own harshest critics! *Do not write yourself off.* Frequently, all is not lost. Don't let your performance dip on the next cases because you are still reeling from the last. Put mistakes behind you, keep calm and carry on!

Station 1
Abdominal and Respiratory

Clinical mark sheet

Clinical skill	Satisfactory	Unsatisfactory
Physical examination	Correct, thorough, fluent, systematic, professional	Incorrect technique, omits, unsystematic, hesitant
Identifying physical signs	Identifies correct signs Does not find signs that are not present	Misses important signs Finds signs that are not present
Differential diagnosis	Constructs sensible differential diagnosis	Poor differential, fails to consider the correct diagnosis
Clinical judgement	Sensible and appropriate management plan	Inappropriate management Unfamiliar with management
Maintaining patient welfare	Respectful, sensitive Ensures comfort, safety and dignity	Causes physical or emotional discomfort Jeopardises patient safety

Cases for PACES, Third Edition. Stephen Hoole, Andrew Fry and Rachel Davies.
© 2015 John Wiley & Sons, Ltd. Published 2015 by John Wiley & Sons, Ltd.

Chronic liver disease and hepatomegaly

This man complains of weight loss and abdominal discomfort. His GP has referred him to you for a further opinion. Please examine his abdomen.

Clinical signs

SIGNS OF CHRONIC LIVER DISEASE
- **General:** cachexia, icterus (also in acute), excoriation and bruising
- **Hands:** leuconychia, clubbing, Dupuytren's contractures and palmar erythema
- **Face:** xanthelasma, parotid swelling and fetor hepaticus
- **Chest and abdomen:** spider naevi and caput medusa, reduced body hair, gynaecomastia and testicular atrophy (in males)

SIGNS OF HEPATOMEGALY
- Palpation and percussion:
  - Mass in the right upper quadrant that moves with respiration, that you are not able to get above and is dull to percussion
  - Estimate size (finger breadths below the diaphragm)
  - Smooth or craggy/nodular (malignancy/cirrhosis)
  - Pulsatile (TR in CCF)
- Auscultation
  - Bruit over liver (hepatocellular carcinoma)

EVIDENCE OF AN UNDERLYING CAUSE OF HEPATOMEGALY
- Tattoos and needle marks   Infectious hepatitis
- Slate-grey pigmentation   Haemochromatosis
- Cachexia   Malignancy
- Mid-line sternotomy scar   CCF

EVIDENCE OF TREATMENT
- Ascitic drain/tap sites
- Surgical scars

EVIDENCE OF DECOMPENSATION
- **A**scites: shifting dullness
- **A**sterixis: 'liver flap'
- **A**ltered consciousness: encephalopathy

Discussion

CAUSES OF HEPATOMEGALY
The **big three:**
Cirrhosis (alcoholic)
Carcinoma (secondaries)
Congestive cardiac failure
Plus: **I**nfectious (HBV and HCV)
          Immune (PBC, PSC and AIH)
          Infiltrative (amyloid and myeloproliferative disorders)

INVESTIGATIONS
- Bloods: FBC, clotting, U&E, LFT and glucose
- Ultrasound scan of abdomen
- Tap ascites (if present)

IF CIRRHOTIC
- Liver screen bloods:
  - Autoantibodies and immunoglobulins (PBC, PSC and AIH)
  - Hepatitis B and C serology
  - Ferritin (haemochromatosis)
  - Caeruloplasmin (Wilson's disease)
  - α-1 antitrypsin
  - Autoantibodies and immunoglobulins (PBC)
  - AFP (hepatocellular carcinoma)
- Hepatic synthetic function: INR (acute) and albumin (chronic)
- Liver biopsy (diagnosis and staging)
- ERCP (diagnose/exclude PSC)

IF MALIGNANCY
- Imaging: CXR and CT abdomen/chest
- Colonoscopy/gastroscopy
- Biopsy

COMPLICATIONS OF CIRRHOSIS
- Variceal haemorrhage due to portal hypertension
- Hepatic encephalopathy
- Spontaneous bacterial peritonitis

CHILD-PUGH CLASSIFICATION OF CIRRHOSIS
Prognostic score based on bilirubin/albumin/INR/ascites/encephalopathy

	Score	1 year survival
A:	5–6	100%
B:	7–9	81%
C:	10–15	45%

CAUSES OF ASCITES
- **C**irrhosis (80%)
- **C**arcinomatosis
- **C**CF

TREATMENT OF ASCITES IN CIRRHOTICS
- Abstinence from alcohol
- Salt restriction
- Diuretics (aim: 1 kg weight loss/day)
- Liver transplantation

CAUSES OF PALMAR ERYTHEMA
- Cirrhosis
- Hyperthyroidism
- Rheumatoid arthritis
- Pregnancy
- Polycythaemia

CAUSES OF GYNAECOMASTIA

- Physiological: puberty and senility
- Kleinfelter's syndrome
- Cirrhosis
- Drugs, e.g. spironolactone and digoxin
- Testicular tumour/orchidectomy
- Endocrinopathy, e.g. hyper/hypothyroidism and Addison's

AUTOANTIBODIES IN LIVER DISEASE

- Primary biliary cirrhosis (PBC): antimitochondrial antibody (M2 subtype) in 98%, increased IgM
- Primary sclerosing cholangitis (PSC): ANA, anti-smooth muscle may be positive
- Autoimmune hepatitis (AIH): anti-smooth muscle, anti-liver/kidney microsomal type 1(LKM1) and occasionally ANA may be positive (pattern helps classify)

Haemochromatosis

This 52-year-old man was referred after a diagnosis of diabetes mellitus was made by his GP. Please examine him and discuss further investigations.

Clinical signs
- Increased skin pigmentation (slate-grey colour)
- Stigmata of chronic liver disease
- Hepatomegaly

SCARS
- Venesection
- Liver biopsy
- Joint replacement
- Abdominal rooftop incision (hemihepatectomy for hepatocellular carcinoma)

EVIDENCE OF COMPLICATIONS
- **Endocrine:** 'bronze diabetes' (e.g. injection sites), hypogonadism and testicular atrophy
- **Cardiac:** congestive cardiac failure
- **Joints:** arthropathy (pseudo-gout)

Discussion

INHERITANCE
- Autosomal recessive on chromosome 6
- **HFE** gene mutation: regulator of gut iron absorption
- Homozygous prevalence 1:300, carrier rate 1:10
- Males affected at an earlier age than females – protected by menstrual iron losses

PRESENTATION
- Fatigue and arthritis
- Chronic liver disease
- Incidental diagnosis or family screening

INVESTIGATION
- ↑ Serum ferritin
- ↑ Transferrin saturation
- Liver biopsy (diagnosis + staging)
- Genotyping

And consider:
• Blood glucose	Diabetes
• ECG, CXR, ECHO	Cardiac failure
• Liver ultrasound, α-fetoprotein	Hepatocellular carcinoma (HCC)

TREATMENT
- Regular venesection (1 unit/week) until iron deficient, then venesect 1 unit, 3–4 times/year
- Avoid alcohol
- Surveillance for HCC

FAMILY SCREENING (1ST DEGREE RELATIVES AGED > 20 YEARS)
- Iron studies (ferritin and TSAT)

If positive:

- Liver biopsy
- Genotype analysis

PROGNOSIS
- 200 × increased risk of HCC if cirrhotic
- Reduced life expectancy if cirrhotic
- Normal life expectancy without cirrhosis + effective treatment

Splenomegaly

This man presents with tiredness and lethargy. Please examine his abdominal system and discuss your diagnosis.

Clinical signs

GENERAL
- Anaemia
- Lymphadenopathy (axillae, cervical and inguinal areas)
- Purpura

ABDOMINAL
- Left upper quadrant mass that moves inferomedially with respiration, has a notch, is dull to percussion and you cannot get above nor ballot
- Estimate size
- Check for hepatomegaly

UNDERLYING CAUSE

	Haematological and infective
Lymphadenopathy	
Stigmata of chronic liver disease	Cirrhosis with portal hypertension
Splinter haemorrhages, murmur, etc.	Bacterial endocarditis
Rheumatoid hands	Felty's syndrome

Discussion

CAUSES
- Massive splenomegaly (>8 cm):
  - Myeloproliferative disorders (**CML** and **myelofibrosis**)
  - Tropical infections (**malaria**, visceral leishmaniasis: kala-azar)
- Moderate (4–8 cm):
  - Myelo/lymphoproliferative disorders
  - Infiltration (Gaucher's and amyloidosis)
- Tip (<4 cm):
  - Myelo/lymphoproliferative disorders
  - Portal hypertension
  - Infections (EBV, infective endocarditis and infective hepatitis)
  - Haemolytic anaemia

INVESTIGATIONS
- Ultrasound abdomen

Then if:

- **Haematological:**
  - FBC and film
  - CT chest and abdomen
  - Bone marrow aspirate and trephine
  - Lymph node biopsy
- **Infectious:**
  - Thick and thin films (malaria)
  - Viral serology

INDICATIONS FOR SPLENECTOMY
- Rupture (trauma)
- Haematological (ITP and hereditary spherocytosis)

SPLENECTOMY WORK-UP
- Vaccination (ideally 2/52 prior to protect against encapsulated bacteria):
  - Pneumococcus
  - Meningococcus
  - *Haemophilus influenzae* (Hib)
- Prophylactic penicillin: (lifelong)
- Medic alert bracelet

Renal enlargement

This woman has been referred by her GP for investigation of hypertension. Please examine her abdomen.

Clinical signs

PERIPHERAL
- Blood pressure: **hypertension**
- Arteriovenous fistulae (thrill and bruit), tunnelled dialysis line
- Immunosuppressant 'stigmata', e.g. Cushingoid habitus due to steroids, gum hypertrophy with ciclosporin

ABDOMEN
- Palpable kidney: ballotable, can get above it and moves with respiration
- Polycystic kidneys: both may/should be palpable, and can be grossly enlarged (will feel 'cystic', or nodular)
- Iliac fossae: scar with (or without!) transplanted kidney
- Ask to dip the urine: proteinuria and haematuria
- Ask to examine the external genitalia (varicocele in males)

ASSOCIATED CONDITIONS
- Hepatomegaly: polycystic kidney disease
- Indwelling catheter: obstructive nephropathy with hydronephrosis
- Peritoneal dialysis catheter/scars

Discussion

CAUSES OF UNILATERAL ENLARGEMENT
- Polycystic kidney disease (other kidney not palpable or contralateral nephrectomy – flank scar)
- Renal cell carcinoma
- Simple cysts
- Hydronephrosis (due to ureteric obstruction)

CAUSES OF BILATERAL ENLARGEMENT
- Polycystic kidney disease
- Bilateral renal cell carcinoma (5%)
- Bilateral hydronephrosis
- Tuberous sclerosis (renal angiomyolipomata and cysts)
- Amyloidosis

INVESTIGATIONS
- U&E
- Urine cytology
- Ultrasound abdomen ± biopsy
- IVU
- CT if carcinoma is suspected
- Genetic studies (ADPKD)

Autosomal dominant polycystic kidney disease:
- Progressive replacement of normal kidney tissue by cysts leading to renal enlargement and renal failure (5% of end-stage renal failure in UK)
- Prevalence 1:1000
- Genetics: 85% *ADPKD1* chromosome 16; 15% *ADPKD2* chromosome 4

- Present with:
  - Hypertension
  - Recurrent UTIs
  - Abdominal pain (bleeding into cyst and cyst infection)
  - Haematuria
- End-stage renal failure by age 40–60 years (earlier in *ADPKD1* than *2*)
- Other organ involvement:
  - Hepatic cysts and hepatomegaly (rarely liver failure)
  - Intracranial Berry aneurysms (neurological sequelae/craniotomy scar?)
  - Mitral valve prolapse
- Genetic counselling of family and family screening; 10% represent new mutations
- Treatment: nephrectomy for recurrent bleeds/infection/size, dialysis and renal transplantation

The liver transplant patient
Please examine this man's abdomen.

Clinical signs
• Scars:

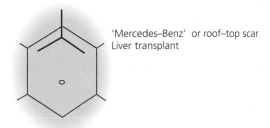

'Mercedes–Benz' or roof–top scar
Liver transplant

• Evidence of chronic liver disease

REASON FOR LIVER TRANSPLANTATION
• Slate-grey pigmentation   Haemochromatosis
• Other autoimmune disease   PBC
• Tattoos and needle marks   Hepatitis B, C

EVIDENCE OF IMMUNOSUPPRESSIVE MEDICATION
• Ciclosporin: gum hypertrophy and hypertension
• Steroids: Cushingoid appearance, thin skin, ecchymoses

Discussion
TOP THREE REASONS FOR LIVER TRANSPLANTATION
• Cirrhosis
• Acute hepatic failure (hepatitis A and B, paracetamol overdose)
• Hepatic malignancy (hepatocellular carcinoma)

SUCCESS OF LIVER TRANSPLANTATION
• 80% 1-year survival
• 70% 5-year survival

CAUSES OF GUM HYPERTROPHY
• Drugs: ciclosporin, phenytoin and nifedipine
• Scurvy
• Acute myelomonocytic leukaemia
• Pregnancy
• Familial

SKIN SIGNS IN (ANY) TRANSPLANT PATIENTS
• **Malignancy**
    ○ Dysplastic change (actinic keratoses)
    ○ Squamous cell carcinoma (100 × increased risk and multiple lesions)
    ○ Basal cell carcinoma and malignant melanoma (10 × increased risk)
• **Infection:**
    ○ Viral warts
    ○ Cellulitis

The renal patient
Please examine this man's abdomen.

Clinical signs
- Stigmata:
  - Arms: arteriovenous fistula(e) – currently working (thrill), being used (thrill and dressings), or failed
  - Neck: tunneled dialysis line (or previous lines; scars in the root of the neck and over the chest wall)
  - Abdomen:

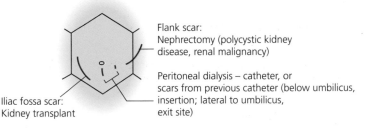

Flank scar:
Nephrectomy (polycystic kidney disease, renal malignancy)

Peritoneal dialysis – catheter, or scars from previous catheter (below umbilicus, insertion; lateral to umbilicus, exit site)

Iliac fossa scar:
Kidney transplant

- Fluid status (leg oedema)

THREE THINGS TO CONSIDER IN ALL RENAL PATIENTS
1. **Underlying reason for renal failure**
   - Polycystic kidneys: ADPKD
   - Visual impairment, fingerprick marks, injection sites/pump, etc.: diabetes
   - Sclerodactyly, typical facies: systemic sclerosis
   - Rheumatoid hands, nodules: rheumatoid arthritis
   - (Hepato)splenomegaly: amyloidosis
   - Other organ transplantation (liver/heart/lungs): calcineurin inhibitor nephrotoxicity
   - Ungual fibromata, adenoma sebaceum, polycystic kidneys: tuberous sclerosis
2. **Current treatment modality**
   - Haemodialysis: working fistula, tunneled neck lines, arteriovenous grafts
   - Peritoneal dialysis: abdominal catheter
   - Functioning transplant: no evidence of other current dialysis access (in use)
3. **Complications of past/current treatment**
   - Side effects of treatment for the underlying disease: Cushingoid appearance from steroids (glomerulonephritis)
   - Side effects of immunosuppressive treatment in transplant patients:
     - Fine tremor (tacrolimus)
     - Steroid side effects
     - Gum hypertrophy (ciclosporin)
     - Hypertension (ciclosporin, tacrolimus)
     - Skin damage and malignancy (especially ciclosporin and azathioprine)
   - Scars from previous access for dialysis, failed transplant(s)

KIDNEY-PANCREAS TRANSPLANTATION
Consider if:

- Lower midline abdominal incision, with a palpable kidney in an iliac fossa (but no overlying scar)

- Evidence of previous diabetes (e.g. visual impairment)
- Patients are often younger (most commonly transplanted in 30s–40s)

Discussion

TOP THREE CAUSES FOR RENAL TRANSPLANTATION
- Glomerulonephritis
- Diabetic nephropathy
- Polycystic kidney disease (ADPKD)

PROBLEMS FOLLOWING TRANSPLANTATION
- **Rejection:** acute or chronic
- **Infection secondary to immunosuppression:**
  - *Pneumocystis carinii*
  - CMV
- **Increased risk of other pathology:**
  - Skin malignancy
  - Post-transplant lymphoproliferative disease
  - Hypertension and hyperlipidaemia causing cardiovascular disease
- **Immunosuppressant drug side effects/toxicity:**
  - Ciclosporin nephrotoxicity
- **Recurrence of original disease**
- **Chronic graft dysfunction**

SUCCESS OF RENAL TRANSPLANTATION
- 90% 1-year graft survival
- 50% 10-year graft survival (better with live-related donor grafts)

Pulmonary fibrosis

Examine this patient's respiratory system, she has been complaining of progressive shortness of breath.

Clinical signs
- Clubbing, central cyanosis and tachypnoea
- Fine end-inspiratory crackles (like Velcro® which do not change with coughing)
- Signs of associated autoimmune diseases, e.g. rheumatoid arthritis (hands), SLE and systemic sclerosis (face and hands)
- Signs of treatment, e.g. Cushingoid from steroids
- Discoloured skin (grey) – amiodarone
- Unless there are any associated features then describe your findings as pulmonary fibrosis, which is a clinical description pending further differentiation following investigations

Discussion

INVESTIGATION
- **Bloods:** ESR, rheumatoid factor and ANA
- **CXR:** reticulonodular changes; loss of definition of either heart border; small lungs
- **ABG:** type I respiratory failure
- **Lung function tests:**
  - $FEV_1/FVC > 0.8$ (restrictive)
  - Low TLC (small lungs)
- Reduced TLco and K_{co}
- **Bronchoalveolar lavage:** main indication is to exclude any infection prior to immunosuppressants plus if lymphocytes > neutrophils indicate a better response to steroids and a better prognosis (sarcoidosis)
- **High-resolution CT scan:** distribution helps with diagnosis; bibasal subpleural honeycombing typical of UIP; widespread ground glass shadowing more likely to be non-specific interstitial pneumonia often associated with autoimmune disease; if apical in distribution then think of sarcoidosis, ABPA, old TB, hypersensitivity pneumonitis, Langerhan's cell histiocytosis.
- Lung biopsy (associated morbidity ~7%)

TREATMENT
- Immunosuppression if likely to be inflammatory; i.e. non-specific interstitial pneumonia e.g. steroids: combination of steroids and azathioprine no longer used following results of PANTHER trial which showed increased morbidity on this combination
- Pirfenidone (an antifibrotic agent) - for UIP when FEV_1 50–80% predicted (NICE recommended)
- N-acetyl cycsteine – free radical scavenger
- Single lung transplant
- NB: Beware single lung transplantation patient – unilateral fine crackles and contralateral thoracotomy scar with normal breath sounds

PROGNOSIS
- Very variable: depends on aetiology
- Highly cellular with ground glass infiltrate – responds to immunosuppression: 80% 5-year survival

- Honeycombing on CT – no response to immunosuppression: 80% 5-year mortality
- There is an increased risk of bronchogenic carcinoma

CAUSES OF BASAL FIBROSIS
- Usual interstitial pneumonia (UIP)
- Asbestosis
- Connective tissue diseases
- Aspiration

Bronchiectasis

This 60-year-old woman presents to your clinic with a persistent cough. Please examine her and discuss your findings.

Clinical signs

General: Cachexia and tachypnoea

Hands: Clubbing

Chest: Mixed character crackles that alter with coughing. Occasional squeaks and wheeze. Sputum + + + (look in the pot!)

- **Cor pulmonale:** SOA, raised JVP, RV heave, loud P_2
- **Yellow nail syndrome:** yellow nails and lymphoedema

Discussion

INVESTIGATION

- Sputum culture and cytology
- CXR: tramlines and ring shadows
- **High-resolution CT thorax:** 'signet ring' sign (thickened, dilated bronchi larger than the adjacent vascular bundle)

FOR A SPECIFIC CAUSE

- **Immunoglobulins:** hypogammaglobulinaemia (especially IgG_2 and IgA)
- *Aspergillus* **RAST or skin prick testing:** ABPA (upper lobe)
- **Rheumatoid serology**
- **Saccharine ciliary motility test** (nares to taste buds in 30 minutes): Kartagener's
- **Genetic screening:** cystic fibrosis
- History of inflammatory bowel disease

CAUSES OF BRONCHIECTASIS

- **Congenital:** Kartagener's and cystic fibrosis
- **Childhood infection:** measles and TB
- **Immune OVER activity:** allergic bronchopulmonary aspergillosis (ABPA); inflammatory bowel disease associated
- **Immune UNDER activity:** hypogammaglobulinaemia; CVID
- **Aspiration:** chronic alcoholics and GORD; localized to right lower lobe

TREATMENT

- Physiotherapy – active cycle breathing
- Prompt antibiotic therapy for exacerbations
- Long-term treatment with low dose azithromycin three times per week
- Bronchodilators/inhaled corticosteroids if there is any airflow obstruction
- Surgery is occasionally used for localized disease

COMPLICATIONS OF BRONCHIECTASIS

- Cor pulmonale
- (Secondary) amyloidosis (Dip urine for protein)
- Massive haemoptysis (mycotic aneurysm)

Old tuberculosis

Please examine this man's respiratory system.

Clinical signs
- Chest deformity and absent ribs; thoracoplasty scar
- Tracheal deviation towards the side of the fibrosis (traction)
- Reduced expansion
- Dull percussion but present tactile vocal fremitus
- Crackles and bronchial breathing

Discussion
HISTORICAL TECHNIQUES
- **Plombage:** insertion of polystyrene balls into the thoracic cavity
- **Phrenic nerve crush:** diaphragm paralysis
- **Thoracoplasty:** rib removal; lung not resected
- Apical lobectomy
- Recurrent medical pneumothoraces
- Streptomycin was introduced in the 1950s. It was the first drug shown to be beneficial in a randomized controlled trial

SERIOUS SIDE EFFECTS OF TB DRUGS
- **Isoniazid**   Peripheral neuropathy (Rx Pyridoxine) and hepatitis
- **Rifampicin**   Hepatitis and increased contraceptive pill metabolism
- **Ethambutol**   Retro-bulbar neuritis and hepatitis
- **Pyrazinamide**   Hepatitis

Prior to treating TB, check baseline liver function tests and visual acuity. Tell the patient the following:

1. Look at the whites of your eyes every morning. If yellow, stop the tablets and ring the TB nurse that morning.
2. Notice colours – if red becomes less bright than you expect ring the TB nurse that day.
3. You may develop tingling in your toes – continue with the tablets but tell the doctor at your next clinic visit.
4. Your secretions will turn orange/red. This is because of a dye in one of the tablets. If you wear contact lenses they will become permanently stained and should not be worn.
5. If you are on the OCP, it may fail. Use barrier contraception.

CAUSES OF APICAL FIBROSIS: 'TRASHE'
- **T**B
- **R**adiation
- **A**nkylosing spondylitis/ABPA
- **S**arcoidosis
- **H**istoplasmosis/Histiocytosis X
- **E**xtrinsic allergic alveolitis (now referred to as hypersensitivity pneumonitis)

Surgical respiratory cases

Please examine this man who initially presented to doctors with a cough and weight loss.

Lobectomy

CLINICAL SIGNS

- Reduced expansion and chest wall deformity
- Thoracotomy scar: same for either upper or lower lobe
- Trachea is central
- Lower lobectomy: dull percussion note over lower zone with absent breath sounds
- Upper lobectomy: may have normal examination or may have a hyper-resonant percussion note over upper zone with a dull percussion note at base where the hemidiaphragm is elevated slightly

INVESTIGATION

- CXR: maybe no overt abnormality apparent other than slight raised hemidiaphragm; remember that the right hemidiaphragm should be higher than the left in health
- CT chest: loss of a lobe with associated truncation of bronchus or pulmonary vessels

Pneumonectomy

CLINICAL SIGNS

- Thoracotomy scar (indistinguishable from thoracotomy scar performed for a lobectomy)
- Reduced expansion on side of the pneumonectomy
- Trachea deviated towards the side of the pneumonectomy
- Dull percussion note throughout the hemithorax
- Absent tactile vocal fremitus beneath the thoracotomy scar
- Bronchial breathing in the upper zone with reduced breath sound throughout remainder of hemithorax (bronchial breathing is due to transmitted sound from major airways)

DISCUSSION

- CXR: complete white out on side of pneumonectomy
- Pneumonectomy space fills with gelatinous material within a few weeks of the operation

Lung transplantation
Signal lung transplant

- Clinical signs: thoracotomy scar; normal exam on side of scar; may have clinical signs on opposite hemithorax
- Indications for 'dry lung' conditions: COPD; pulmonary fibrosis

Double lung transplant

- Clinical signs: clamshell incision – from the one axilla along the line of the lower ribs, up to the xiphisternum to the other axilla
- Indications: 'wet lung' conditions: CF, bronchiectasis or pulmonary hypertension

Chronic obstructive airways disease
Please examine this patient's chest; he has a chronic chest condition.

Clinical signs
- Inspection: nebulizer/inhalers/sputum pot, dyspnoea, central cyanosis and pursed lips
- CO_2 retention flap, bounding pulse and tar-stained fingers
- Hyper-expanded
- Percussion note resonant with loss of cardiac dullness
- Expiratory polyphonic wheeze (crackles if consolidation too) and reduced breath sounds at apices
- Cor pulmonale: raised JVP, ankle oedema, RV heave; loud P_2 with pansystolic murmur of tricuspid reurgitation
- COPD does not cause clubbing: therefore, if present consider bronchial carcinoma or bronchiectasis

Discussion
- Spectrum of disease with airway obstruction (with or without sputum production); can be low FEV_1 at one end and emphysema with low O_2 sats but normal spirometry at the other
- Degree of overlap with chronic asthma, although in COPD there is less reversibility (<15% change in FEV_1 post-bronchodilators)

CAUSES
- Environmental: smoking and industrial dust exposure (apical disease)
- Genetic: α_1-antitrypsin deficiency (basal disease)

INVESTIGATIONS
- **CXR:** hyper-expanded and/or pneumothorax
- **ABG:** type II respiratory failure (low PaO_2 high $PaCO_2$)
- **Bloods:** high WCC (infection), low α_1-antitrypsin (younger patients/FH+), low albumin (severity)
- **Spirometry:** low FEV_1, FEV_1/FVC < 0.7 (obstructive)
- **Gas transfer:** low T_LCO

TREATMENT
- **Medical** – depends on severity **(GOLD classification):**
  - **Smoking cessation** is the single most beneficial management strategy
  - Cessation clinics and nicotine replacement therapy
  - Long-term oxygen therapy (LTOT)
  - Pulmonary rehabilitation
  - Mild (FEV_1 >80) – beta-agonists
  - Moderate (FEV_1 <60%) – tiotropium plus beta-agonists
  - Severe (FEV_1 <40%) or frequent exacerbations – above plus inhaled corticosteroids; although avoid if patient has ever had an episode of pneumonia (TORCH trial)
  - Exercise
  - Nutrition (often malnourished)
  - Vaccinations - pneumoccoal and influenza

- **Surgical** (careful patient selection is important)
  - Bullectomy (if bullae >1 L and compresses surrounding lung)
  - Endobronchial valve placement
  - Lung reduction surgery: only suitable for a few patient with heterogeneous distribution of emphysema
  - Single lung transplant

LONG-TERM OXYGEN THERAPY (LTOT)
- **Inclusion criteria:**
  - Non-smoker
  - PaO_2 <7.3 kPa on air
  - $PaCO_2$ that does not rise excessively on O_2
  - If evidence of cor pulmonale, PaO_2 <8 kPa
- 2–4 L/min via nasal prongs for at least 15 hours a day
- Improves average survival by 9 months

TREATMENT OF AN ACUTE EXACERBATION
- Controlled O_2 via Venturi mask monitored closely
- Bronchodilators
- Antibiotics
- Steroids 7 days

PROGNOSIS
COPD patients with an acute exacerbation have 15% in-hospital mortality

DIFFERENTIAL OF A WHEEZY CHEST
- Granulomatous polyarteritis (previously Wegner's): saddle nose; obliterative bronchiolitis
- Rheumatoid arthritis: wheeze secondary to obliterative bronchiolitis
- Post-lung transplant: obliterative bronchiolitis as part of chronic rejection spectrum

Pleural effusion

This patient has been breathless for 2 weeks. Examine his respiratory system to elucidate the cause.

Clinical signs

- Asymmetrically reduced expansion
- Trachea or mediastinum displaced away from side of effusion
- **Stony** dull percussion note
- Absent tactile vocal fremitus
- Reduced breath sounds
- Bronchial breathing above (aegophony)

SIGNS THAT MAY INDICATE THE CAUSE

- **Cancer:** clubbing; lymphadenopathy; mastectomy (breast cancer being a very common cause of pleural effusion)
- **Congestive cardiac failure:** raised JVP; peripheral oedema
- **Chronic liver disease:** leuconychia, spider naevi gynaecomastia
- **Chronic renal failure:** arteriovenous fistula
- **Connective tissue disease:** rheumatoid hands; butterfly rash of SLE

CAUSES OF A DULL LUNG BASE

- **Consolidation:** bronchial breathing and crackles
- **Collapse:** tracheal deviation towards the side of collapse and reduced breath sounds
- Previous lobectomy = reduced lung volume
- **Pleural thickening:** signs are similar to a pleural effusion but with normal tactile vocal fremitus; may have three scars suggestive of previous VATS pleuradesis
- **Raised hemidiaphragm** ± hepatomegaly

Discussion

CAUSES

Transudate (protein <30 g/L)	Exudate (protein >30 g/L)
Congestive cardiac failure	Neoplasm: 1° or 2°
Chronic renal failure	Infection
Chronic liver failure	Infarction
	Inflammation: RA and SLE

Pleural aspiration (exudate)

- **Protein:** effusion albumin/plasma albumin >0.5 (Light's criteria)
- **LDH:** effusion LDH/plasma LDH >0.6
- **Empyema:** an exudate with a low glucose and pH <7.2 is suggestive

Empyema

- A collection of pus within the pleural space
- Most frequent organisms: anaerobes, staphylococci and Gram-negative organisms
- Associated with bronchial obstruction, e.g. carcinoma, with recurrent aspiration; poor dentition; alcohol dependence

TREATMENT

- Pleural drainage and IV antibiotics intrapleural DNAse plus TPA (MIST 2 Trial)
- Surgical decortication

Lung cancer

Please examine this patient who has had a 3-month history of chronic cough, malaise and weight loss.

Clinical signs
- Cachectic
- Clubbing and tar-stained fingers
- Lymphadenopthy: cervical and axillary
- Tracheal deviation: towards (collapse) or away (effusion) from the lesion
- Reduced expansion
- Percussion note dull (collapse/consolidation) or stony dull (effusion)
- Absent tactile vocal fremitus (effusion); increased vocal resonance (collapse/consolidation)
- Auscultation:
  - Crackles and bronchial breathing (consolidation/collapse)
  - Reduced breath sounds; absent tactile fremitus (effusion)
- **Hepatomegaly or bony tenderness:** metastasis
- **Treatment:**
  - Lobectomy scar
  - **Radiotherapy:** square burn and **tattoo**
- **Complications:**
  - **Superior vena cava obstruction:** suffused and oedematous face and upper limbs, dilated superficial chest veins and stridor
  - **Recurrent laryngeal nerve palsy:** hoarse with a 'bovine' cough
  - **Horner's sign and wasted small muscles of the hand (T1):** Pancoast's tumour
  - **Endocrine:** gynaecomastia (ectopic βHCG)
  - **Neurological:** Lambert–Eaton myasthenia syndrome, peripheral neuropathy, proximal myopathy and paraneoplastic cerebellar degeneration
  - **Dermatological:** dermatomyositis (heliotrope rash on eye lids and purple papules on knuckles (Gottron's papules associated with a raised CK) and acanthosis nigricans

Discussion

TYPES
- Squamous 35%, small (oat) 24%, adeno 21%, large 19% and alveolar 1%

MANAGEMENT
1. Diagnosis of a mass:
   - **CXR:** collapse, mass and hilar lymphadenopathy
   - **Volume acquisition CT thorax** (so small tumours are not lost between slices) with contrast
2. Determine cell type:
   - **Induced sputum cytology**
   - **Biopsy** by **bronchoscopy** (central lesion and collapse) or **percutaneous needle** CT guided (peripheral lesion; $FEV_1 >1\,L$))
3. Stage (**CT/bronchoscopy/endobronchial ultrasound guided biopsy/ mediastinoscopy/thoracoscopy/PET**):
   - **Non-small cell carcinoma (NSCLC): TNM staging to assess operability**
   - Small cell carcinoma (SCLC): limited or extensive disease
4. Lung function tests for operability assessment:
   - Pneumonectomy contraindicated if $FEV_1 < 1.2\,L$
5. Complications of the tumour:
   - Metastasis: ↑ LFTs, ↑ Ca^{++}, ↓ Hb
   - NSCLC: ↑ PTHrP → ↑ Ca^{++}
   - SCLC: ↑ ACTH, SIADH → Na^+ ↓

TREATMENT
- **NSCLC:**
  - **Surgery:** lobectomy or pneumonectomy
  - **Radiotherapy:** single fractionation (weekly) versus hyper-fractionation (daily for 10 days)
  - **Chemotherapy:** benefit unknown; EGFR Positive – erlotinib
- **SCLC:**
  - **Chemotherapy:** benefit with six courses

Multidisciplinary approach
PALLIATIVE CARE
- Dexamethasone and radiotherapy for brain metastasis
- SVCO: dexamethasone plus radiotherapy or intravascular stent
- Radiotherapy for haemoptysis, bone pain and cough
- Chemical pleurodesis for effusion – talc; tetracycline no longer used
- Opiates for cough and pain

Cystic fibrosis

Please examine this young man's chest and comment on what you find.

Clinical signs

- Inspection: small stature, **clubbed**, tachypnoeic, sputum pot (purulent++)
- Hyperinflated with reduced chest expansion
- **Coarse crackles** and wheeze (bronchiectatic)
- **Portex reservoir** (Portacath®) under the skin or **Hickman line/scars** for long-term antibiotics plus PEG for malabsorption

Discussion

GENETICS

- Incidence of 1/2500 live births
- Autosomal recessive chromosome 7q
- Gene encodes CFTR (Cl⁻channel)
- Commonest and most severe mutation is the deletion Δ508/ Δ508 (70%)

PATHOPHYSIOLOGY

Secretions are thickened and block the lumens of various structures:

- Bronchioles → bronchiectasis
- Pancreatic ducts → loss of exocrine and endocrine function
- Gut → distal intestinal obstruction syndrome (DIOS) in adults
- Seminal vesicles → male infertility
- Fallopian tubes – reduced female fertility

INVESTIGATIONS

- Screened at birth: low immunoreactive trypsin (heel prick)
- Sweat test: $Na^+ > 60$ mmol/L (false-positive in hypothyroidism and Addison's)
- Genetic screening

TREATMENT

- **Physiotherapy:** postural drainage and active cycle breathing techniques
- Prompt antibiotics for intercurrent infections
- Pancrease® and fat-soluble vitamin supplements
- Mucolytics (DNAse)
- Immunizations
- Double lung transplant (50% survival at 5 years)
- Gene therapy is under development

PROGNOSIS

Median survival is 35 years but is rising. Poor prognosis if becomes infected with *Burkholderia cepacia*

Pneumonia
This patient has been acutely unwell for 3 days, with shortness of breath and a productive cough. Please examine his chest.

Clinical signs
- Tachypnoea, O_2 mask, sputum pot (rusty sputum associated with *pneumococcus*)
- Reduced expansion
- Dull percussion note
- Focal coarse crackles, increased vocal resonance and bronchial breathing
- Ask for the temperature chart
- If dull percussion note with absent tactile vocal fremitus, think parapneumonic effusion/ empyema

Discussion
INVESTIGATION
- **CXR:** consolidation (air bronchogram), abscess and effusion
- **Bloods:** WCC, CRP, urea, atypical serology (on admission and at day 10) and immunoglobulins
- **Blood** (25% positive) and **sputum cultures**
- **Urine:**
  - ○ *Legionella* antigen (in severe cases)
  - ○ *Pneumococcal* antigen
  - ○ Haemoglobinuria (*mycoplasma* causes cold agglutinins → haemolysis)

COMMUNITY ACQUIRED PNEUMONIA (CAP)
- Common organisms:
  - ○ **Streptococcus pneumoniae** 50%
  - ○ **Mycoplasma pneumoniae** 6%
  - ○ *Haemophilus influenzae* (especially if COPD)
  - ○ *Chlamydia pneumoniae*.
- Antibiotics:
  - ○ 1st line: penicillin *or* cephalosporin ı macrolide

SPECIAL CONSIDERATIONS
- **Immunosuppressed:**
  - ○ Fungal — Rx Amphotericin
  - ○ Multi-resistant mycobacteria
  - ○ *Pneumocystis carinii* — Rx Cotrimoxazole/Pentamidine
  - ○ CMV — Rx Ganciclovir
- **Aspiration** (commonly posterior segment of right lower lobe):
  - ○ Anaerobes — Rx + Metronidazole
- **Post-influenza:**
  - ○ *Staph. aureus* — Rx + Flucloxacillin

SEVERITY SCORE FOR PNEUMONIA: CURB-65 (2/5 IS SEVERE)
- **C**onfusion
- **U**rea >7
- **R**espiratory rate >30
- **B**P systolic <90 mm Hg or diastolic <60 mm Hg
- **Age >65**

Severe CAP should receive high-dose IV antibiotics initially plus level 2 care (HDU/ITU)

PREVENTION
Pneumovax II® to high-risk groups, e.g. chronic disease (especially nephrotic and asplenic patients) and the elderly

COMPLICATIONS
- Lung abscess (*Staph. aureus*, *Klebsiella*, anaerobes)
- Para-pneumonic effusion/empyema
- Haemoptysis
- Septic shock and multi-organ failure

Station 2
History Taking

Clinical mark sheet

Clinical skill	Satisfactory	Unsatisfactory
Clinical communication skills	Elicits full history Systematic, fluent, professional Assesses impact of symptoms Provides a clear and accurate clinical information	Omits important history Unsystematic, unpractised, unprofessional, unstructured Uses jargon Inaccurate information provided
Managing patients' concerns	Seeks, detects and addresses concerns Listens, empathetic Confirms understanding	Over-looks concerns Poor listening Not empathetic Does not check understanding
Differential diagnosis	Constructs sensible differential diagnosis	Poor differential, fails to consider the correct diagnosis
Clinical judgement	Sensible and appropriate management plan	Inappropriate management Unfamiliar with management
Maintaining Patient Welfare	Respectful, sensitive Ensures comfort, safety and dignity	Causes physical or emotional discomfort Jeopardises patient safety

Cases for PACES, Third Edition. Stephen Hoole, Andrew Fry and Rachel Davies.
© 2015 John Wiley & Sons, Ltd. Published 2015 by John Wiley & Sons, Ltd.

Introduction and advice

Prior to entering the room you will have 5 minutes to read the 'GP referral letter'. Then you will take a history from the patient in front of both examiners. At the end of 14 minutes the patient will leave the room and you will have a minute to gather your thoughts before 5 minutes of discussion with the examiners. You should not present the history back to them, but rather produce a problem list to discuss.

The format of this section will teach you how to do this.

Surprisingly more candidates fail this station than any other. Yet it is often ignored in examination preparation.

There are essentially two types of history you will encounter. In one the patient presents with a collection of symptoms and you must attempt to reach a diagnosis. In the other the patient has a chronic disease where the diagnosis is clear but you must review previous investigation, treatments and search out possible complications. Examples of both of these will be presented.

Take note of the following points. **Many of these are specifically mentioned on the examiner's mark sheet**.

- **Use preparation time wisely**

Before you enter the room you will have 5 minutes to read the GP letter. You will be provided with blank paper, which you may take into the room. Use this time to note down a written structure for the interview with key points that you must not forget when the adrenaline is flowing! For example, in a diagnosis question a written list of differentials will prompt you to ask appropriate questions to support or refute each. This helps you reach the final diagnosis in a logical and systematic way and scores more marks than an apparently jumbled sequence of questions.

- **Take a complete history**

Systems review, past medical history, family history, drug history, smoking and alcohol are all specifically mentioned on the mark sheet. You will lose points for neglecting them. Actors may be primed to give you certain information only if specifically questioned upon it.

- **Explore psychosocial issues**

The impact of the condition on his or her relationships, family and job is crucial and in the examination, patients will probably not volunteer this unless asked. In most cases this should feature on your subsequent list of problems.

- **Attempt to develop a rapport**

The way you interact with the patient is assessed. Attempt to put them at ease. Respond appropriately to things they tell you – do not say 'good' after hearing about their recent bereavement! Appear sympathetic if required. Maintain appropriate levels of eye contact. Balance open and closed questions.

- **Review information with patient**

Again this is specifically mentioned on the mark sheet but is often neglected. Tell the patient you would like to check you have the story straight. Not only does this confirm the facts but may well clarify things to you that had not been apparent before.

- **Adhere to a time structure**

There will be a clock in the room that will be easily visible to you. You have 14 minutes with the patient. You will throw away marks if you do not finish within time. Clearly, each case will vary but as a rough guide aim to spend 5 minutes on the presenting complaint, 4 minutes on past medical, drug and family histories and 4 minutes on social history. This leaves you 1 minute to review information with the patient and then a further minute to get your thoughts straight for the discussion.

- **Generate a problem list**

By now you should have generated a list of the main issues pertinent to the case. This may be a single diagnosis but may be an extensive list including medical problems, social problems and concerns or complaints about treatment. This will form the crux of your discussion.

• **Think ahead about your discussion**

This is likely to involve questions on further investigation and management, so anticipate this as you go along.

Scoring well on this station requires good examination technique. It is rather different to the history you take daily at work and it is also the station that most candidates underestimate during preparation for the examination.

What follows are 12 typical examples that we suggest you practise in small groups. The cases are introduced with a GP letter. We also include a briefing to be read only by the person role-playing the patient. At the end there is a suggested problem list to compare with your own along with likely discussion points. You must practise these with strict timings and ideally with others observing. You must be used to taking a complete and logical history and having your problem list ready for discussion at the 15-minute point.

As in the examination the cases are deliberately varied. Some focus on a single medical problem while others involve multiple medical and social issues. The cases are based on real PACES cases.

Case 1

Dear Dr,

I would be grateful for your opinion on this 48-year-old lady who was diagnosed with rheumatoid arthritis 5 years ago. She has noticed increased swelling of her ankles for the last 2 months and has 3+ proteinuria on dipstick urinalysis today.

Case 2

Dear Dr,

I would be grateful for your assessment of this 55-year-old man with poorly controlled diabetes. He has previously been reluctant to attend a diabetic clinic. He is currently taking oral hypoglycaemic medication and bendroflumethiazide. I feel he may need to start insulin soon. I calculated his body mass index today at 36. His last HbA1C was 97 mmol/mol (11%).

Case 3

Dear Dr,

This 26-year-old female attended my surgery today complaining of difficulty walking that had come on over a few days. On examination she has a markedly ataxic gait but no other abnormality. She has no significant past medical history and takes only simple analgesia for headaches. I would be grateful for your urgent assessment.

Case 4

Dear Dr,

Thank you for seeing this 35-year-old teacher urgently. I am concerned she has had a pulmonary embolus. She developed central pleuritic chest pain during the course of yesterday; however, she has felt generally unwell for a week. She was on the combined oral contraceptive pill until 1 year ago. She currently takes fluoxetine for depression and nifedipine for Raynaud's syndrome.

On examination she was a little breathless. Pulse 100; BP 170/100. Chest clear.

Case 5

Dear Dr,

I would be grateful if you would see this 22-year-old language student who has had persistent diarrhoea since returning from Russia 2 months ago. Several of her friends on her trip also had diarrhoea whilst abroad but unlike them her symptoms have not settled with antibiotics.

Case 6
Dear Dr,

I would be grateful for your opinion on this 78-year-old man who has recurrent dizzy spells and on two occasions he has blacked out at home. He had a pacemaker inserted 2 years ago following an episode of heart block, which complicated an anterior myocardial infarction. I wondered if the pacemaker was malfunctioning, though a recent check was satisfactory. His only other medical history is hypertension. In the surgery today his pulse was 70 regular and BP 135/85.

Case 7
Dear Dr,

Thank you for seeing this 56-year-old businessman who came to see me because his wife was concerned he looked a bit yellow. Apart from looking a little jaundiced there was no abnormality on physical examination today. His liver function tests are deranged with an elevated ALT and bilirubin. Otherwise he is well and only takes bendroflumethiazide for hypertension.

Case 8
Dear Dr,

Thank you for seeing this 30-year-old shop assistant who complains of amenorrhoea for 6 months. She has a history of manic depression for which she is under psychiatric review but is currently well and off medication. A pregnancy test was negative. Her body mass index was calculated at 25.

Case 9
Dear Dr,

We have had this 30-year-old man on our asthma clinic registry since he was a teenager although he has never been very diligent about attending his appointments. However, he now complains that his breathing has been getting very much worse over the last few months and his symptoms are not controlled with Ventolin and Becotide. I would be grateful for your opinion.

Case 10
Dear Dr,

Many thanks for seeing this 20-year-old man who feels increasingly fatigued and unwell. On examination he has bilateral cervical lymphadenopathy, which has been increasing for at least 2 months. There are no nodes elsewhere and there is no other abnormality on physical examination.

Case 11
Dear Dr,

This 66-year-old female has suffered two episodes of transient loss of consciousness. Apart from these episodes she is in good health. Her medical history includes a myocardial infarct 4 years ago and mastectomy 9 years ago. She takes aspirin 75 mg od, atenolol 50 mg od and enalapril 10 mg od. She is a non-smoker. Physical examination of neurological and cardiovascular systems was normal with blood pressure 110/65 mm Hg. An ECG showed sinus rhythm 60 bpm and inferior q-waves from her previous MI.

Case 12

Dear Dr,

I would be grateful for your advice on this 40-year-old male who was diagnosed with antiphospholipid syndrome following a pulmonary embolus 3 years ago. Long-term anticoagulation with warfarin (target INR 2.5) was advised then. Recently he seems increasingly resistant to warfarin requiring doses of 15 mg daily. Despite this his INR is frequently subtherapeutic. In addition, on one occasion he has been admitted via A&E for INR > 20. I have checked his antiphospholipid antibody levels which remain greatly elevated and would be grateful for you advise on his management.

Case 1
Briefing for patient
You are 48 years old.

You were diagnosed with rheumatoid arthritis 5 years ago after developing painful, swollen wrists and hands. Your GP took some blood tests and referred you to a rheumatologist for a specialist opinion. You were treated with an injection of steroids and then started on methotrexate. This has kept your disease under reasonable control since then.

You have had a few more problems with your hands and knee joints over the past few months. When prompted, you state that you have dealt with these by taking courses of over-the-counter NSAIDs.

You first noticed that your ankles were a bit more swollen a couple of months ago, but didn't think much of it at the time. They have progressively worsened since then and you have had problems getting your shoes on. They are not painful – not like your arthritis – but they are uncomfortable. They do seem to be less swollen in the morning, but in the last week you have noticed that your face is puffy when you first get up. You don't have any other systemic symptoms, and your breathing is normal. If pushed, you would agree that your urine is more frothy than previously.

You saw your GP about this new problem a couple of weeks ago. She told you that you had some 'fluid retention', likely to be related to the recent hot weather. You went back again this week as the problem worsened, and were asked to provide a urine sample on this occasion. She has given you a new 'water tablet', but it doesn't appear to have had any effect.

Your current medications are methotrexate once a week, folic acid, occasional ibuprofen and paracetamol, plus a new prescription of furosemide.

You deny any previous kidney problems.

You worked as a secretary until you had your two children 10 years ago, but not since. You are happily married and your husband is a solicitor.

Your parents are both fit and well as are your children and brother.

You have never smoked and drink an occasional glass of wine.

Problem list
- Background of **rheumatoid arthritis**, with reasonable control on a **disease-modifying anti-rheumatic drug** (DMARD), methotrexate.
- Now presents with peripheral oedema, facial oedema and frothy urine, suggesting a diagnosis of **nephrotic syndrome**.
- No other complications of rheumatoid suggested by the history, e.g. pulmonary or pleural involvement or anaemia.

Discussion
- Systemic complications of rheumatoid arthritis.
- Diagnosis of the nephrotic syndrome (clinical criteria) and further investigation, including role of renal biopsy.
- Potential causes of the nephrotic syndrome.
- Treatment of rheumatoid disease and the use of DMARDs.

Case 2
Briefing for patient

You are 55 years old.

Diabetes was diagnosed 10 years ago and initially treated with diet alone. When this was not successful, tablets were introduced by your GP and the doses gradually increased.

You currently take metformin 850 mg tds, gliclazide 160 mg bd and bendroflumethiazide 2.5 mg daily. You generally take your tablets as prescribed because your wife nags you to.

Your eyesight is good and you have regular checks at an ophthalmologist.

You are aware of the importance of looking after your feet and have no foot ulcers. Other than high blood pressure you have no other medical problems.

Your cholesterol has never been checked.

You work as an HGV driver.

You smoke 30 cigarettes a day.

You drink very little alcohol.

You are aware of that your diet is not good and that you are rather overweight.

You take very little exercise.

You are happily married with two children aged 15 and 18.

Diabetes runs in your family – father and both brothers.

Your father had a heart attack at the age of 55 and your brother recently had a bypass operation. This worries you although you have had no heart problems to your knowledge.

Problem list

- **Poorly controlled diabetes** on maximal oral hypoglycaemic treatment.
- **Obesity** will exacerbate insulin resistance and is likely to be made worse by starting insulin. Weight loss will improve glycaemic control as well as reducing cardiovascular risk.
- **High risk for ischaemic heart disease**. Smoking must be addressed. Check lipids and if necessary treat. Hypertension should be aggressively controlled ideally with an ACE inhibitor, e.g. ramipril, which has additional cardio-protection properties.
- Starting insulin would result in **loss of HGV licence**.

Discussion

- Management: he is likely to need insulin but this will result in the loss of his job. A serious attempt to lose weight should first be made. This may improve glycaemic control sufficiently to delay the need for insulin. Reduction of cardiac risk is a major component of his management.
- Complications of diabetes, e.g. retinopathy, neuropathy, nephropathy and atherosclerosis, their identification and management.
- Evidence to support the use of ACE inhibitors in diabetes, e.g. HOPE trial.

Case 3
Briefing for patient

You are a 26-year-old student who is normally fit and well.

For the last week you have had difficulty walking and keep stumbling over to the right. As a result you have been unable to play hockey this week. Your friends say you look as if you are drunk. The severity varies a little from day to day but was most severe two nights ago. If specifically asked, this followed a long soak in the bath.

Your speech is normal and your arms seem OK. You have not had a fit or a blackout. You get headaches when you are tired or stressed. The headaches are eased with paracetamol. The headaches have perhaps been a little worse recently. They come on late in the day and have never occurred in the morning on waking. They are not associated with nausea.

This time last year your speech went funny for a few days while on holiday, but it resolved before you saw a doctor. It is difficult to describe it but it sounded funny and slightly slurred.

If specifically asked, you may volunteer the fact that your vision became quite blurred in your right eye for about a week several months ago. The eye also felt painful at the time. Then it came back to normal. Around the same time you had a few episodes when you wet yourself in bed. You were very embarrassed about this but it has not recurred.

You have no other medical problems.

You take no medications at all.

You drink 5–6 glasses of wine at weekends but not during the week.

You do not smoke.

Both parents are fit and well. You are an only child.

Problem list

- **Truncal ataxia** with a background of symptoms suggesting **optic neuritis**, dysarthria and urinary incontinence. The **relapsing/remitting** nature of these symptoms, separated in time and location, in a young adult is virtually diagnostic of **multiple sclerosis**. This is supported further by the presence of Uthoff's phenomenon (worsening of symptoms by heat – in this case a hot bath).
- The headaches sound like simple **tension headaches** and do not require further investigation.

Discussion

- Investigation and management of multiple sclerosis
- Differential diagnosis of headaches
- Socio-economic impact of chronic disability

Case 4
Briefing for patient
You are a 35-year-old teacher.

You have felt generally unwell and run down for several months.

You have felt hot and shivery for a few weeks. Yesterday you noticed pain in the centre of your chest. The pain is sharp and grating. It hurts when you breathe in deeply. The only position you are comfortable in is sitting upright and last night you could not sleep lying down because of the pain. Exertion and eating do not affect the pain.

You are not short of breath. Your legs do not swell up; you have not been on an airline recently, and have not been immobilized either.

For years you have had Raynaud's syndrome treated with nifedipine by the GP. Your hands get very cold and turn white, blue and then red if you do not wear gloves in winter. Recently your wrists and hand joints are intermittently painful to the point that it is sometimes hard to write at work.

Two years ago you were admitted with sharp pains in left side of chest and suspicion of a clot on the lung. However, the VQ scan was normal and you were discharged.

If asked, you have no skin rash currently; however, you react badly to the sun and easily get burned especially across your face.

You have felt very depressed recently and have been off work intermittently for 3 months. You feel too run down to work at the moment. Anti-depressants are not really working. You work as a relief teacher and are not paid if you do not work. The lack of income is a major problem at home as your husband has recently been made redundant.

You do not smoke but admit to drinking too much – roughly a bottle of wine per day.

Your parents are both alive and well, and you do not have any siblings. You have one healthy 4-year-old boy (you had three miscarriages in your 20s).

Problem list
- The presenting problem is suggestive of **acute pericarditis**.
- She also describes a background of non-specific ill health with **Raynaud's** phenomenon, **polyarthritis, photosensitivity** and previous **pleurisy**.
- This collection of symptoms suggests an underlying connective tissue disease such as **SLE**.
- Remember also the **hypertension** noted by the GP. Possible renal involvement.
- She feels **depressed**, perhaps due to the symptoms of her disease or perhaps caused directly by SLE.
- The disease is causing significant **work, family** and **financial problems**.
- Her **alcohol** intake is above the recommended safe levels.

Discussion
- Management of acute pericarditis
- Complications of SLE
- Further investigation and management of SLE
- Given her miscarriages anti-phospholipid syndrome might be discussed

Case 5
Briefing for patient

You are a 22-year-old university language student who returned 2 months ago from a year in Russia as part of your course. Your final examinations are in 3 months time.

About 3 months ago while in Russia, you developed diarrhoea. This has continued since then although not as bad. In Russia, the diarrhoea was occurring up to 10 times a day; now it occurs around three times a day. You usually have little warning and are occasionally incontinent. You are very embarrassed about talking about this.

On direct questioning, there is red blood mixed in with the diarrhoea normally preceded by cramping lower abdominal pains. Often you have the sensation of needing to go but are unable to produce anything when you try to open your bowels.

You have not lost weight nor had any fevers. You ate Russian food for the whole year and it had not previously upset you. A couple of your friends developed diarrhoea. They were told it was giardiasis and they got better with antibiotics. Your GP has tried this but it has not really helped.

In the past you have been fit and active although troubled a little recently by lower back pain. This started about a year ago. It is worse in the mornings and usually eases within a few hours of getting up. Sometimes you take ibuprofen when it is bad. No other joints are painful. In Russia you also developed unexplained painful bruising on your shins, which gradually went away after a few weeks. You thought nothing of it and would not mention this unless asked about skin rashes.

You do not smoke. You drink in moderation. You live in a hall of residence and are currently studying for your examinations. The only medicine you ever take is ibuprofen for backache. Your mother, father and sister are all fit and healthy.

Problem list

- Persistent bloody diarrhoea and tenesmus is suggestive of **ulcerative colitis**.
- A history compatible with both **sacroilitis** and **erythema nodosum** is evident and associated with ulcerative colitis.
- Giardiasis, whilst common in Eastern Europe and Russia, does not cause bloody diarrhoea. Other infectious causes of bloody diarrhoea, e.g. *Shigella* and *Salmonella*, should be excluded by stool microscopy and culture.
- There is anxiety about incontinence during her imminent examinations.

Discussion

- Differential diagnosis and investigation of bloody diarrhoea
- Management of colitis

Case 6
Briefing for patient
You are 78 years old.

Over the last 2 months you have suffered from recurrent dizzy spells. Sometimes these are bad enough that you have to sit or lie down for a few minutes before it resolves. The room does not actually spin around but you feel very light-headed and faint. Last week you actually collapsed in your bedroom after getting up to pass water in the night. You did not hurt yourself nor did you wet yourself and once you took it steady you were able to get to the toilet. You were not out for long and knew exactly what had happened afterwards. A similar thing has happened before while you were washing up. As it starts, you sometimes get tunnel vision and feel sweaty before you collapse.

You have no chest pain, palpitations or breathlessness either at rest or on exertion. The attacks are not related to moving your head around and you have no ear problems. There have been no problems with your speech or limbs. These attacks have never occurred while sitting or lying down. If you stand up too quickly the symptoms occur.

In the past you have had a heart attack and needed a pacemaker afterwards. This was checked 3 weeks ago and was said to be fine. The blackouts you had then were different, occurring without warning whilst sitting or standing. You have mild heart failure but this has been well controlled lately and you are able to walk to the shops easily. You have had high blood pressure in the past but recently this has been lower according to your GP. Your ramipril dose was increased at a hospital appointment about 3 months ago.

You live alone. You normally cope fine, but are currently very worried about what would happen if you had a fall and hurt yourself as there is no one nearby that you could phone. You do not smoke or drink.

Problem list
- The story is suggestive of **postural hypotension** and the ACE inhibitor is the likely culprit.
- Excluded other causes of dizziness and collapse:
  - **Cardiac:** arrhythmia/aortic stenosis
  - **Neurological:** posterior circulation TIAs/epilepsy
  - **Other:** micturition syncope, carotid sinus sensitivity and vasovagal
- The patient lives alone and falls jeopardize his independence. Perhaps a 'lifeline' alarm system would be appropriate.

Discussion
- Falls and syncope in the elderly
- Side effects of ACE inhibitors

Case 7
Briefing for patient
You are 56 years old.

Recently your wife has commented you look jaundiced which is why you went to the doctor. Looking back you have been feeling generally tired for 6 months or more - but put this down to the stress of your job - and have lost about 9 lb in weight. Your skin has been intermittently very itchy and you have been scratching a lot. You have had some very minor vague aches in the right side of your abdomen but nothing severe. You have not had a fever. There have been no other symptoms.

You have travelled abroad only to France recently. You have never been outside Europe. You have not been in contact with anyone jaundiced.

You have never used IV drugs although did smoke cannabis as a student. You have no tattoos.

You drink two or three pints of beer at weekends but have never drunk heavily.

You do not smoke.

You are happily married with two children. Apart from your wife you have had no other sexual partners. You have had some problems with erectile dysfunction recently, but don't mention this unless specifically asked.

You work as a salesman and have no exposure to sewage, drains or outdoor water.

Your GP started you on bendroflumethiazide 2 years ago for hypertension. You take no other over-the-counter or herbal medication.

Your father had liver problems and died when you were in your early teens, and your younger brother has recently been diagnosed with diabetes.

Problem list
- The family history of liver disease and diabetes, plus his erectile dysfunction, is strongly suggestive of hereditary haemochromatosis.
- It is important to explore other causes of abnormal liver function tests, in particular alcohol, medications and risks for chronic viral hepatitis.

Discussion
- Investigation of a jaundiced patient
- Investigation of abnormal LFTs.
- Diagnosis, genetics and management of hereditary haemochromatosis.
- Management of the patient with cirrhosis from any cause.

Case 8
Briefing for patient
You are a 30-year-old shop assistant.

Over the last year your periods have become progressively more irregular and you have now not had a period at all for 6 months. Otherwise you feel well. You do not think you could be pregnant as you have used barrier contraception with your current partner and two pregnancy tests have been negative.

You exercise normally but not excessively and eat a normal diet.

You have no symptoms of hot or cold intolerance and do not suffer with palpitations or tremor and your bowels are normal. You do not suffer from dizziness or faints or excessive thirst.

You do not suffer with indigestion.

You do not have headaches.

You do not have a problem with your vision, but recently crashed your car because 'a car came out of no-where'.

You have noticed that you have been lactating over the past few weeks. You are embarrassed but also quite worried about this and would only divulge this personal information if asked in a direct but sensitive way.

You had an operation on your neck 3 years ago for high calcium levels, which was diagnosed after you had a small kidney stone.

You saw a psychiatrist around the same time for depression and take Prozac intermittently when you feel like it. You have taken no other medication.

Your mother and sister are fit and well. Your father died in his 50s from a bleeding ulcer for which he had previously had surgery. You think he also had an operation on his neck at some stage.

You do not smoke and rarely drink alcohol.

You are happily married and keen to start a family in the near future.

Problem list
- Amenorrhoea and galactorrhoea are suggestive of a pituitary adenoma including a **prolactinoma**.
- **Dopamine antagonists**, e.g. anti-psychotics, can cause hyperprolactinaemia but rarely SSRIs, and in this case their prescription preceded the symptoms by 2 years.
- **Other pituitary** function appears to be normal.
- Crashing the car may have been due to **bi-temporal hemianopia**.
- The background of **hyperparathyroidism** ('bones, **stones**, abdominal groans and **psychic moans**') and the **family history** suggestive of hyperparathyroidism and recurrent peptic ulceration (gastrinoma) suggests **multiple endocrine neoplasia type I (MEN I)**.
- She wants to have children but is currently likely to be **infertile**.

Discussion
- Investigation of a pituitary adenoma and management
- Details of MEN I
- Causes of secondary amenorrhoea. Referral to a fertility specialist and genetic counselling may be needed once the pituitary lesion has been treated

Case 9
Briefing for patient

You are 30 years old and were first diagnosed with asthma as a teenager.

Until recently your symptoms have never been very severe and consisted of cough at night and intermittent wheezy days. Ventolin® has always been very effective. You did not go to your GP asthma clinic because your breathing was never very bad and all they did was nag you about smoking. You have never been admitted to hospital with asthma.

Over the last few months, however, your breathing has been getting steadily worse. Your asthma is particularly bad in the evenings with cough, wheezing and breathlessness, which prevent you from going out when severe. Now your breathing is bad most nights. You have not coughed up any sputum and have not had a fever. You have had no pain in your chest.

There have been days when your chest is fine and on a recent family holiday to France you had no symptoms at all and your exercise tolerance was unlimited.

There is nothing at home that seems to precipitate the asthma. You have no pets or birds. Your sister has a cat that has always made your asthma worse when you visit her house but you have not been there recently.

You work in a car factory on a production line. You are not involved in the spray painting although it does happen nearby. You do not wear a mask. The spray sometimes causes a runny nose and cough but does not seem to cause the wheezing as this only comes on later in the afternoons and evening. However, your symptoms do seem to be a bit better at weekends and were much better when away on holiday for a week.

You have been doing this job for a year now and enjoy working and earning good money. Previously you were unemployed for nearly 2 years and you had to go on the dole to support your wife and two small children. You almost got a divorce during this time and you blame 'money problems' for almost wrecking your marriage.

You are currently using a salbutamol inhaler. You have a Becotide inhaler but rarely use this as it makes very little difference.

You smoke five cigarettes per day and are trying to cut down. You do not drink alcohol. Your parents and brother are fit and have no respiratory problems.

Problem list

- Deterioration in asthma with a temporal relationship to work suggests **occupational asthma**. It is not uncommon for onset of symptoms to be delayed for a few hours after exposure. The history of relief of symptoms during holiday is typical. Spray painting is one of the commonest causes of occupational asthma.
- **Poor compliance and asthma education** are also playing a role.
- Continued smoking is a problem.
- **Financial problems** and difficulty finding work are relevant.

Discussion

- Might involve further investigation of asthma by peak-flow diaries to confirm the relationship between work and asthma.
- Occupational asthma management may also be covered (the only effective treatment is avoidance of precipitant).
- Employees with occupational asthma are eligible for industrial injury benefit.

Case 10
Briefing for patient
You are a 20-year-old English student.

For the last 4 months you have been troubled by recurrent coughs and colds. You have intermittently coughed up yellow sputum but no blood. You now feel you have no energy and are completely unable to study. You noticed some lumps in your neck recently, which have been enlarging.

If asked:

You have not had a sore throat or a rash.

You have not travelled abroad other than to Spain 2 years ago.

You have no contact with TB.

You have no pets.

You have lost about 14 lb in weight over the last 2 months.

You have had to change bedclothes almost daily due to drenching night sweats.

You have not used IV drugs.

You are homosexual and have had one partner for a year. Neither of you have had an HIV test.

You used to drink a lot of alcohol but have recently found that you feel awful when you drink and your neck hurts a lot so you have abstained totally for the last month.

You smoke 20 cigarettes per day.

You have never been ill before nor taken any medication.

Your family members are all fit and well.

Problem list
- Lymphadenopathy, weight loss and drenching night sweats are suggestive of lymphoma, in particular **Hodgkin's disease**
- Other differentials include:
  - Infection: **HIV, glandular fever** and **TB**
  - Inflammatory: sarcoid and connective tissue disease
  - Solid tumour: **adenocarcinoma** and melanoma (smokes but young age)
- Drugs

Discussion
- Differential diagnosis
- Investigations of lymphadenopathy and diagnosis of Hodgkin's disease: Reed–Sternberg cells on lymph node biopsy
- Management

Case 11
Briefing for patient

You are 66 years old. Three weeks ago you collapsed in the kitchen whilst preparing breakfast. Your husband was upstairs at the time and heard a crash followed by some unusual noises. When he came down you initially looked blue and were foaming at the mouth. He could not rouse you or move you. There was some blood because you had banged your head on the table and the teapot was smashed. Your husband fetched a neighbour who helped you onto the sofa as you had come round a little by then. You do not actually remember the collapse itself and do not even remember moving to the sofa. You only really became aware of what had happened later on about the time your daughter arrived – this must have been about 2 hours later. By then you felt OK but very tired and somewhat embarrassed about all the fuss. The following day you felt completely normal again.

If asked you would admit that you also wet yourself during the attack but are embarrassed and would not volunteer this information. You did not bite your tongue. You had a mild headache afterwards but this is probably due to banging your head when you collapsed. You had no unusual symptoms or warning of any kind prior to the attack. You did not feel unwell or dizzy prior to the episode and you had no breathlessness or chest pain. You have not had any of these symptoms at any stage. You have had no weakness of arms or legs and no speech or visual problem.

Two weeks later a very similar episode occurred.

You suffered a heart attack 4 years ago at which time you had bad chest pain and went to hospital. Since then you have been on tablets for your heart; these have caused you no side effects and you have had no further heart problems. You had a mastectomy 9 years ago for a small breast cancer. The operation was successful and you were given the 'all clear' and discharged from clinic several years ago.

You do not smoke. You drink very little alcohol. You take no medication or drugs of any kind other than those prescribed by your GP. You are a retired school teacher. Your husband still works full time. Your GP mentioned that you might have to stop driving for a few weeks but this would be extremely inconvenient for you at the moment as you have just had your first grandchild and your daughter is relying on you to help out with the baby several days each week. She lives in a small village with few links to public transport.

Problem list

- The history is suggestive of a **generalized seizure** with post-ictal state.
- The possible differential diagnosis of **malignant ventricular arrhythmia following her MI** and **postural hypotension/bradycardia** secondary to cardiac medication should be explored.
- The past history of breast cancer makes it important to rule out metastases and planned investigations should address this.
- The social implications of **driving restriction** to this patient should be recognized.

Discussion

- Investigation and treatment of first generalized seizure
- DVLA driving restrictions (see Station 4, Driving restrictions)
- Emergency management of status epilepticus

Case 12
Briefing for the patient
About 3 years ago you collapsed with chest pain and breathlessness and were diagnosed with a blood clot in the lung. You spent 2 weeks in hospital and were told you were lucky to survive. You started warfarin tablets at that point. You had not had any clots prior to this. You have had one more clot in your leg 8 months ago. Your leg swelled up and was painful and a scan showed a clot in the thigh. At the time you were on warfarin but your levels were said to be very low. You have not had any clots since. You have never had a stroke. No one in your family has had a blood clot.

Your INR levels were good at first but for the last year you have had to have a lot of blood tests and they always seem too high or too low and the GP keeps changing the dose. You are supposed to run between 2 and 3. Recently the level was over 20 and you had to spend a night in hospital. You have not had any abnormal bleeding.

You know that it is important to take your warfarin but you do sometimes forget. You usually take it in the evening but sometimes in the mornings depending on when you remember. Recently you have missed more doses but you do not really believe the amount you take has much effect on the INR because the levels do not bear much relation to whether you take it or not.

You used to work as a night watchman but have been out of regular employment since the factory closed a year ago. Now you do ad hoc work when you can get it which can be day or night shifts. You drink quite heavily. You admit you drink too much and a number of your friends have commented on this which irritates you. If pushed you would admit you sometimes drink a bottle of vodka every one to two days sometimes starting in the morning. The time you were admitted to hospital with high levels of warfarin followed a period of very heavy drinking and was around the time your marriage broke up. You had also had a chest infection and had been on antibiotics. You now live alone. You have no children. You have a very poor diet except for when you stay with your mother who makes you eat healthily for a few weeks. She also thinks you are depressed and gives you a tablet that she says works for her for depression. She buys it from the chemist and it does not require a prescription – you take it sometimes as it can't do any harm. She also gives you multi-vitamin tablets that you take sometimes.

Problem list
- Antiphospholipid syndrome with recurrent venous thromboembolism including a life-threatening PE and a recurrence on warfarin.
- Erratic INR due to:
  - Poor **compliance** with warfarin prescription
  - **Alcoholism**
  - Poor **diet** with intermittent vitamin supplementation leading to fluctuating vitamin K intake
  - **Drug interactions** – erythromycin contributed to his admission with high INR. Over the counter St John's Wort may increase warfarin metabolism
  - The **antiphospholipid syndrome** itself may also cause an erratic INR.

Discussion
- Duration of warfarin treatment for single or recurrent PE/DVT
- Screening for prothrombotic states
- Management of anticoagulated patients who require invasive procedures, e.g. liver biopsy to exclude cirrhosis
- Emergency reversal of anticoagulation
- Alternatives to warfarin for long-term anticoagulation – low molecular weight heparin and the novel oral anticoagulants. Home INR monitoring may result in better compliance.

Station 3
Cardiology and Neurology

Clinical mark sheet

Clinical skill	Satisfactory	Unsatisfactory
Physical examination	Correct, thorough, fluent, systematic, professional	Incorrect technique, omits, unsystematic, hesitant
Identifying physical signs	Identifies correct signs Does not find signs that are not present	Misses important signs Finds signs that are not present
Differential diagnosis	Constructs sensible differential diagnosis	Poor differential, fails to consider the correct diagnosis
Clinical judgement	Sensible and appropriate management plan	Inappropriate management Unfamiliar with management
Maintaining patient welfare	Respectful, sensitive Ensures comfort, safety and dignity	Causes physical or emotional discomfort Jeopardises patient safety

Cases for PACES, Third Edition. Stephen Hoole, Andrew Fry and Rachel Davies.
© 2015 John Wiley & Sons, Ltd. Published 2015 by John Wiley & Sons, Ltd.

Aortic stenosis

This patient presents with increasing dyspnoea. Examine his cardiovascular system to elucidate the cause.

Clinical signs
- Slow rising, low volume pulse
- Narrow pulse pressure
- Apex beat is **s**ustained in **s**tenosis (**HP: h**eaving **p**ressure-loaded)
- Thrill in aortic area (right sternal edge, second intercostal space)
- Auscultation

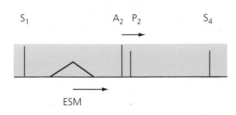

A crescendo-decrescendo, ejection systolic murmur (ESM) loudest in the aortic area during expiration and radiating to the carotids.

Severity:
soft and delayed A_2 due to immobile leaflets and prolonged LV emptying, delayed (not loud) ESM, fourth heart sound S_4.

Discussion
EVIDENCE OF COMPLICATIONS
- **Endocarditis:** splinters, Osler's nodes (finger pulp), Janeway lesions (palms), Roth spots (retina), temperature, splenomegaly and haematuria
- **Left ventricular dysfunction:** dyspnoea, displaced apex and bibasal crackles
- **Conduction problems: acute**, endocarditis; **chronic**, calcified aortic valve node

DIFFERENTIAL DIAGNOSIS
- HOCM
- VSD
- Aortic sclerosis: normal pulse character and no radiation of murmur
- Aortic flow: high output clinical states e.g. pregnancy or anaemia

CAUSES OF AS
Congenital: bicuspid
Acquired: **A**ge (senile degeneration and calcification); **S**treptococcal (rheumatic)

ASSOCIATIONS
- Coarctation and bicuspid aortic valve
- Angiodysplasia

SEVERITY

Symptom	50% mortality at
Angina	5 years
Syncope	3 years
Breathlessness	2 years

- **Signs**

Auscultation features (see figure), biventricular failure (right ventricular failure is preterminal).

INVESTIGATIONS
- **ECG:** LVH on voltage criteria, conduction defect (prolonged PR interval)
- **CXR:** often normal; calcified valve
- **Echo:** mean gradient: >40 mm Hg aortic (valve area <1.0 cm²) if severe
- **Catheter:** invasive transvalvular gradient and coronary angiography (coronary artery disease often coexists with aortic stenosis)

MANAGEMENT
- **Asymptomatic**
  - None specific, good dental health
  - Regular review: symptoms and echo to assess gradient and LV function
- **Symptomatic**
  - Surgical
    - Aortic valve replacement +/− CABG
    - Operative mortality 3–5% depending on the patient's EuroScore (www.euroscore.org/calc.html)
  - Percutaneous
    - Balloon aortic valvuloplasty (BAV)
    - Transcutaneous aortic valve implantation (TAVI)
      - Transfemoral (or transapical and transaortic)
      - Maybe recommended if high surgical risk (logEuroscore >20%) or inoperable cases (number needed to treat to prevent death at 1 year = 5)

Duke's criteria for infective endocarditis
Major:
- Typical organism in two blood cultures
- Echo: abscess*, large vegetation*, dehiscence*
Minor:
- Pyrexia >38°C
- Echo suggestive
- Predisposed, e.g. prosthetic valve
- Embolic phenomena*
- Vasculitic phenomena (ESR↑, CRP↑)
- Atypical organism on blood culture

Diagnose if the patient has 2 major, 1 major and 2 minor, or 5 minor criteria.
(* plus heart failure/refractory to antibiotics/heart block are indicators for urgent surgery).

Antibiotic prophylaxis is now limited to those with **prosthetic valves, previous endocarditis, cardiac transplants with valvulopathy** and **certain types of congenital heart disease**.

Aortic incompetence

This patient has been referred by his GP with 'a new murmur'. He is asymptomatic. Please examine his cardiovascular system and diagnose his problem.

Clinical signs
- Collapsing pulse (waterhammer pulse) reflecting a wide pulse pressure, e.g. 180/45
- Apex beat is hyperkinetic and displaced laterally (**TV: t**hrusting **v**olume-loaded)
- Thrill in the aortic area
- Auscultation:

S_1 A_2 P_2

Early diastolic murmur (EDM) loudest at the lower left sternal edge with the patient sat forward in expiration.

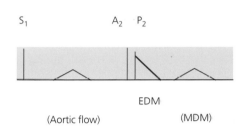

EDM

(Aortic flow)   (MDM)

There may be an aortic flow murmur and a mid-diastolic murmur (MDM) (Austin–Flint) due to regurgitant flow impeding mitral opening.

In severe AR there may be 'free flow' regurgitation and the EDM may be silent.

- **Signs of severity:** collapsing pulse, third heart sound (S_3) and pulmonary oedema
- **Eponymous signs**
  - Corrigan's: visible vigorous neck pulsation
  - Quincke's: nail bed capillary pulsation
  - De Musset's: head nodding
  - Duroziez's: diastolic murmur proximal to femoral artery compression
  - Traube's: 'pistol shot' sound over the femoral arteries

Discussion
CAUSES
- Congenital: bicuspid aortic valve; perimembranous VSD
- Acquired:

	Acute	Chronic
Valve leaflet	Endocarditis	Rheumatic fever
		Drugs: pergolide, slimming agents
Aortic root	Dissection (type A)	Dilatation: Marfan's and hypertension
	Trauma	Aortitis: syphilis, ankylosing spondylitis and vasculitis

OTHER CAUSES OF A COLLAPSING PULSE
- Pregnancy
- Patent ductus arteriosus

- Paget's disease
- Anaemia
- Thyrotoxicosis

INVESTIGATION
- **ECG:** lateral T-wave inversion
- **CXR:** cardiomegaly, widened mediastinum and pulmonary oedema
- **TTE/TOE:**
  Severity: LVEF and dimensions, root size, jet width
  Cause: intimal dissection flap or vegetation
- **Cardiac catheterization:** grade severity aortogram and check coronary patency

MANAGEMENT
Medical
- ACE inhibitors and ARBs (reducing afterload)
- Regular review: symptoms and echo: LVEF, LV size and degree of AR

Surgery
Acute:
- Dissection
- Aortic root abscess/endocarditis (homograft preferably)

Chronic:
Replace the aortic valve when:
- **Symptomatic:** dyspnoea and reduced exercise tolerance (NYHA > II) ***AND/OR***
- **The following criteria are met:**
  1. wide pulse pressure >100 mm Hg
  2. ECG changes (on ETT)
  3. echo: LV enlargement >5.5 cm systolic diameter or EF <50%

Ideally replace the valve prior to significant left ventricular dilatation and dysfunction.

PROGNOSIS
Asymptomatic with EF > 50% – 1% mortality at 5 years.
Symptomatic and all three criteria present – 65% mortality at 3 years.

Mitral stenosis

This patient has been complaining of reduced exercise tolerance. Examine his heart and elucidate the cause of his symptoms.

Clinical signs
- Malar flush
- Irregular pulse if AF is present
- Tapping apex (palpable first heart sound)
- Left parasternal heave if pulmonary hypertension is present or enlarged left atrium
- Auscultation

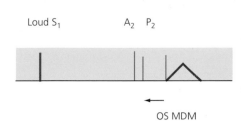

Loud first heart sound. Opening snap (OS) of mobile mitral leaflets opening followed by a mid-diastolic murmur (MDM), which is best heard at the apex, in the left lateral position in expiration with the bell. Presystolic accentuation of the MDM occurs if the patient is in sinus rhythm.

If the mitral stenosis is severe then the OS occurs nearer A_2 and the MDM is longer.

- **Haemodynamic significance**
  Pulmonary hypertension: functional tricuspid regurgitation, right ventricular heave, loud P_2.
  LVF: pulmonary oedema, RVF: sacral and pedal oedema.
- **Endocarditis**
- **Embolic complications:** stroke risk is high if mitral stenosis + AF

Discussion
CAUSES
Congenital: (rare)
Acquired
- **Rheumatic** (commonest)
- Senile degeneration
- Large mitral leaflet vegetation from endocarditis (mitral 'plop' and late diastolic murmur)

DIFFERENTIAL DIAGNOSIS
Left atrial myxoma
Austin–Flint murmur

INVESTIGATION
- **ECG:** p-mitrale (broad, bifid) and atrial fibrillation
- **CXR:** enlarged left atrium (splayed of carina), calcified valve, pulmonary oedema
- **TTE/TOE:** valve area (<1.0 cm² is severe), cusp mobility, calcification and left atrial thrombus, right ventricular failure

MANAGEMENT
- **Medical:** + AF: rate control and oral anticoagulants, diuretics
- **Mitral valvuloplasty:** if pliable, non-calcified with minimal regurgitation and no left atrial thrombus
- **Surgery:** closed mitral valvotomy (without opening the heart) or open valvotomy (requiring cardiopulmonary bypass) or valve replacement

PROGNOSIS
Latent asymptomatic phase 15–20 years; NYHA > II – 50% mortality at 5 years.

RHEUMATIC FEVER
- Immunological cross-reactivity between Group A β-haemolytic streptococcal infection, e.g. *Streptococcus pyogenes* and valve tissue
- **Duckett–Jones diagnostic criteria**
  Proven β-haemolytic streptococcal infection diagnosed by throat swab, rapid antigen detection test (RADT), anti-streptolysin O titre (ASOT) or clinical scarlet fever **plus** 2 major or 1 major and 2 minor:

Major	Minor
Chorea	Raised ESR
Erythema marginatum	Raised WCC
Subcutaneous nodules	Arthralgia
Polyarthritis	Previous rheumatic fever
Carditis	Pyrexia
	Prolonged PR interval

- **Treatment:** Rest, high-dose aspirin and penicillin
- **Prophylaxis:**
  - Primary prevention: penicillin V (or clindamycin) for 10 days
  - Secondary prevention: penicillin V for about 5–10 years

Mitral incompetence
This patient has been short of breath and tired. Please examine his cardiovascular system.

Clinical signs
- Scars: lateral thoracotomy (valvotomy)
- Pulse: AF, small volume
- Apex: displaced and volume loaded
- Palpation: thrill at apex
- Auscultation:

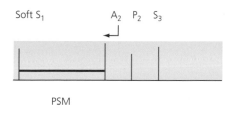

Soft S$_1$ A$_2$ P$_2$ S$_3$

PSM

Pan-systolic murmur (PSM) loudest at the apex radiating to the axilla. Loudest in expiration. Wide splitting of A$_2$P$_2$ due to the earlier closure of A$_2$ because the LV empties sooner.

S$_3$ indicates rapid ventricular filling from LA, and excludes significant mitral stenosis.

- Pulmonary oedema
- Cause: signs of endocarditis (see pages 45–46)
- Severity: left ventricular failure and atrial fibrillation (late). Not murmur intensity
- Other murmurs, e.g. ASD (see page 60)

Discussion
CAUSES
- Congenital (association between cleft mitral valve and primum ASD)
- Acquired:

	Acute	Chronic
Valve leaflets	Bacterial endocarditis	Myomatous degeneration (prolapse)
		Rheumatic
		Connective tissue diseases
		Fibrosis (fenfluramine/pergolide)
Valve annulus		Dilated left ventricle (functional MR)
		Calcification
Chordae/papillae	Rupture	Infiltration, e.g. amyloid
		Fibrosis (post-MI/trauma)

INVESTIGATION
- **ECG:** p-mitrale, atrial fibrillation and previous infarction (Q waves)
- **CXR:** cardiomegaly, enlargement of the left atrium and pulmonary oedema

- **TTE/TOE:**
  Severity: size/density of MR jet, LV dilatation and reduced EF
  Cause: prolapse, vegetations, ruptured papillae, fibrotic restriction and infarction

MANAGEMENT
- **Medical**
  - Anticoagulation for atrial fibrillation or embolic complications
  - Diuretic, β-blocker and ACE inhibitors
- **Percutaneous:** mitral clip device for palliation in inoperative cases of mitral valve prolapse
- **Surgical**
  - Valve repair (preferable) with annuloplasty ring or replacement
  - Aim to operate when symptomatic, prior to severe LV dilatation and dysfunction

PROGNOSIS
- Often asymptomatic for >10 years
- Symptomatic – 25% mortality at 5 years

Mitral valve prolapse
- Common (5%), especially young tall women
- Associated with connective tissue disease, e.g. Marfan's syndrome and HOCM
- Often asymptomatic, but may present with chest pain, syncope and palpitations
- Small risk of emboli and endocarditis
- Auscultation

S_1 EC A_2 P_2 S_3

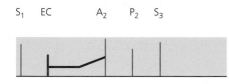

Mid-systolic ejection click (EC). Pan-systolic murmur that gets louder up to A_2.

Murmur is accentuated by standing from a squatting position or during the straining phase of the Valsalva manoeuvre, which reduces the flow of blood through the heart.

Tricuspid incompetence

Examine this patient's cardiovascular system. He has been complaining of abdominal discomfort.

Clinical signs
- Raised JVP with giant CV waves
- Thrill left sternal edge
- Auscultation

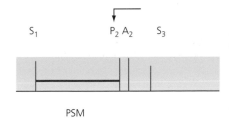

S_1 $P_2 A_2$ S_3

PSM

Pan-systolic murmur (PSM) loudest at the tricuspid area (lower left sternal edge) in inspiration.

Reverse split second heart sound due to rapid RV emptying.

Right ventricular rapid filling gives an S_3.

- Pulsatile liver, ascites and peripheral oedema
- Endocarditis from IV drug abuse: needle marks
- Pulmonary hypertension: RV heave and loud P_2
- Other valve lesions: rheumatic mitral stenosis

Discussion

CAUSES
- **Congenital:** Ebstein's anomaly (atrialization of the right ventricle and TR)
- **Acquired:**
  Acute: infective endocarditis (IV drug user)
  Chronic: functional (commonest), rheumatic and carcinoid syndrome

INVESTIGATION
- ECG: p-pulmonale (large, peaked) and RVH
- CXR: double right heart border (enlarged right atrium)
- TTE: TR jet, RV dilatation

MANAGEMENT
- **Medical:** diuretics, β-blockers, ACE inhibitors and support stockings for oedema
- **Surgical:** valve repair/annuloplasty if medical treatment fails

Pulmonary stenosis

Examine this patient's cardiovascular system. He has had swollen ankles.

Clinical signs
- Raised JVP with giant a waves
- Left parasternal heave
- Thrill in the pulmonary area
- Auscultation

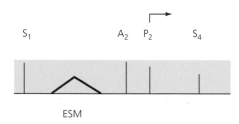

S_1 A_2 P_2 S_4

ESM

Ejection systolic murmur (ESM) heard loudest in the pulmonary area in inspiration.

Widely split second heart sounds, due to a delay in RV emptying.

Severe: inaudible P_2, longer murmur duration obscuring A_2.

- Right ventricular failure: ascites and peripheral oedema
- **Tetralogy of Fallot:** PS, VSD, overriding aorta and RVH (sternotomy scar)
- **Noonan's syndrome:** phenotypically like Turner's syndrome but male sex
- Other murmurs: functional TR and VSD

Discussion
INVESTIGATION
- ECG: p-pulmonale, RVH and RBBB
- CXR: oligaemic lung fields and large right atrium
- TTE: severity (pressure gradient), RV function and associated cardiac lesions

MANAGEMENT
- Pulmonary valvotomy – if gradient >70 mm Hg or there is RV failure
- Percutaneous pulmonary valve implantation (PPVI)
- Surgical repair/replacement

Carcinoid syndrome
- Gut primary with liver metastasis secreting 5-HT into the blood stream
- Toilet-symptoms: diarrhoea, wheeze and flushing!
- Secreted mediators cause right-sided heart valve fibrosis resulting in tricuspid regurgitation and/or pulmonary stenosis
- Rarely a bronchogenic primary tumour or a right-to-left shunt can release 5-HT into the systemic circulation and cause left-sided valve scarring
- Treatment: octreotide or surgical resection

Prosthetic valves: aortic and mitral

This patient has recently been treated for dyspnoea/chest pain/syncope. Please examine his cardio-vascular system.

Clinical signs

• Audible prosthetic clicks (metal) on approach and scars on inspection

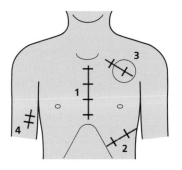

1 Midline sternotomy (CABG, AVR, MVR)
2 Lateral thoracotomy (MVR, mitral valvotomy, coarctation repair, BT shunt)
3 Subclavicular (Pacemaker, AICD)
4 Anticubital fossa (angiography)

Also look in the wrist and groins for angiography scars/bruising and legs for saphenous vein harvest used in bypass grafts.

• Auscultation: don't panic!

Aortic valve replacement

S_1 OC   CC P_2

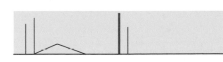

Flow murmur

A metal prosthetic closing click (CC) is heard instead of A_2.
There may be an opening click (OC) and ejection systolic flow murmur.
A bioprosthesetic valve often has normal heart sounds.

Abnormal findings:
AR
Decreased intensity of the closing click (clot or vegetation)

Mitral valve replacement

CC S_2 OC

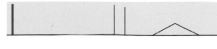

Flow murmur

A metal prosthetic closing click is heard instead of S_1.
An opening click may be heard in early diastole followed by a low-frequency diastolic rumble.

Abnormal findings:
MR
Decreased intensity of the closing click.

• Anticoagulation: bruises (metal valve) and anaemia

Discussion
Choice of valve replacement

	For	Against	Indication
Metal	Durable	Warfarin	Young/on warfarin, e.g. for AF
Porcine	No warfarin	Less durable	Elderly/at risk of haemorrhage

* Operative mortality: 3–5%

LATE COMPLICATIONS
* **Thromboembolus:** 1–2% per annum despite warfarin
* **Bleeding:** fatal 0.6%, major 3%, minor 7% per annum on warfarin
* **Bioprosthetic dysfunction and LVF:** usually within 10 years, can be treated percutaneously (valve-in-valve)
* **Haemolysis:** mechanical red blood cell destruction against the metal valve
* **Infective endocarditis:**
  ○ Early infective endocarditis (<2/12 post-op) can be due to *Staphylococcus epidermidis* from skin
  ○ Late infective endocarditis is often due to *Strep. viridans* by haematogenous spread
  ○ A second valve replacement is usually required to treat this complication
  ○ Mortality of prosthetic valve endocarditis approaches 60%
* **Atrial fibrillation:** particularly if MVR

Implantable devices

This patient has had syncope. Please examine his cardiovascular system.

Clinical signs

- Incisional scar in the infraclavicular position (may be abdominal)
- Palpation demonstrates a pacemaker
- Signs of heart failure: raised JVP, bibasal crackles and pedal oedema
- Medic alert bracelet
- Local infection: red/hot/tender/fluctuant/erosion

Discussion

NICE GUIDANCE

Implantable cardiac defibrillators (ICD)

'Shock box' also delivers anti-tachycardia pacing (ATP) – improves mortality

PRIMARY PREVENTION

- MI > 4 weeks ago (NYHA no worse than class III)
  - ○ LVEF < 35% **and** non-sustained VT **and** positive EP study **or**
  - ○ LVEF < 30% **and** QRSd ≥ 120 milliseconds
- Familial condition with high-risk SCD
  - ○ LQTS, ARVD, Brugada, HCM, complex congenital heart disease

SECONDARY PREVENTION (WITHOUT OTHER TREATABLE CAUSE)

- cardiac arrest due to VT or VF **or**
- haemodynamically compromising VT **or**
- VT with LVEF < 35% (not NYHA IV)

Cardiac resynchronization therapy (CRT) – biventricular pacemakers (BiV)

Extra LV pacemaker lead via the coronary sinus – improves mortality/symptoms
   May be considered if:

- LVEF < 35%
- NYHA II–IV on optimal medical therapy
- Sinus rhythm and QRSd > 150 milliseconds (if LBBB morphology may be >120 milliseconds)

Pericardial disease
Constrictive pericarditis

This man has had previous mantle radiotherapy for lymphoma and has a chronic history of leg oedema, bloating and weight gain.

Clinical signs
- Predominantly right-side heart failure
  - Raised JVP
    - Dominant, brief y-descent due to rapid early ventricular filling and rise in diastolic pressure

Jugular venous pressure waves

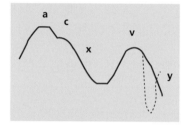

a: atrial systole
c: closure of tricuspid valve
x: movement of atrioventricular ring during ventricular systole
v: filling of the atrium
y: opening of the tricuspid valve

Rapid dominant y-descent due to high RA pressures and an early rise in RV diastolic pressure due to poor pericardial compliance.

  - Kussmaul's sign: paradoxical increase in JVP on inspiration (may need to sit the patient at 90° rather than 45° to observe the JVP meniscus)
  - Pulsus paradoxus:
    - >10 mm Hg drop in systolic pressure in inspiration (not a true paradox as it normally decreases by 2–3 mm Hg!)
  - Auscultation:
    - Pericardial knock – it's not a knock but a high-pitched snap (audible, early S3 due to rapid ventricular filling into a stiff pericardial sac)
  - Ascites, hepatomegaly (congestion) and bilateral peripheral oedema
- Cause:
  - **T**B: cervical lymphadenopathy
  - **T**rauma (or surgery): sternotomy scar, post-MI
  - **T**umour, **T**herapy (radio): radiotherapy tattoos, thoracotomy scar
  - Connective **T**issue disease: rheumatoid hands, SLE signs

Discussion
- Investigation:
  - CXR: pericardial calcification, old TB, sternotomy wires
  - Echo: high acoustic signal from pericardium, septal bounce, reduced mitral flow velocity during inspiration
  - Catheter laboratory:
    - Dip and plateau of the diastolic wave form: square-root sign
    - Equalization of LV and RV diastolic pressures
  - CT: thickened pericardium
- Pathophysiology:
  - Thickened, fibrous capsule reduces ventricular filling and 'insulates' the heart from intrathoracic pressure changes during respiration leading to **ventricular interdependence** – filling of one ventricle reduces the size and filling of the other.

- Treatment:
  - Medical: diuretics and fluid restriction
  - Surgical: pericardial stripping

Differentiating pericardial constriction from restrictive cardiomyopathy is difficult but observing ventricular interdependence (fluctuating LV/RV pressure or MV/TV flow velocities during respiration) is highly diagnostic for constriction!

OTHER COMMON CONGENITAL DEFECTS

Atrial septal defect

This young woman complains of cough and occasional palpitations. Examine her cardiovascular system.

Clinical signs
- Raised JVP
- Pulmonary area thrill
- Auscultation

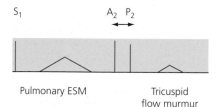

Pulmonary ESM   Tricuspid flow murmur

Fixed split-second heart sounds that do not change with respiration. Pulmonary ejection systolic and mid-diastolic flow murmurs with large left-to-right shunts.

There is no mumur from the ASD itself.

Consider:
- Pulmonary hypertension: RV heave and loud P_2, + cyanosis and clubbing (Eisenmenger's: right-to-left shunt)
- Congestive cardiac failure

Discussion

TYPES
- Primum associated with AVSD and cleft mitral valve) seen in Down's syndrome
- Secundum (commonest)

COMPLICATIONS
- Paradoxical embolus
- Atrial arrhythmias
- RV dilatation

INVESTIGATION
- ECG: RBBB + LAD (primum) or + RAD (secundum); atrial fibrillation
- CXR: small aortic knuckle, pulmonary plethora and double-heart-border (enlarged RA)
- TTE/TOE: site, size and shunt calculation; amenability to closure
- Right heart catheter shunt calculation (not always necessary)

MANAGEMENT
Indications for closure:

- Symptomatic: paradoxical systemic embolism, breathlessness
- Significant shunt: Qp:Qs>1.5:1, RV dilatation

Contraindication for closure:

- Severe pulmonary hypertension and Eisenmenger's syndrome

CLOSURE
- Percutaneous closure device
  - Secundum ASD only, no left atrial appendage thrombus or anomalous pulmonary venous drainage, adequate rim to anchor device
- Surgical patch repair

Ventricular septal defect

This patient has developed sudden shortness of breath. Examine his heart.

Clinical signs
- Thrill at the lower left sternal edge
- Auscultation:

S_1 A_2 P_2

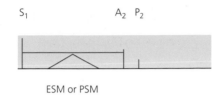

ESM or PSM

Systolic murmur well localized at the left sternal edge with no radiation.
No Audible A_2.

Loudness does not correlate with size (Maladie de Roger: loud murmur due to high-flow velocity through a small VSD).

If Eisenmenger's develops the murmur often disappears as the gradient diminishes.

Extra points
Consider:
- Other associated lesions: AR, PDA (10%), Fallot's tetralogy and coarctation
- Pulmonary hypertension: loud P_2 and RV heave + cyanosis and clubbing (Eisenmenger's)
- Endocarditis

Discussion
CAUSES
- Congenital
- Acquired (traumatic, post-operative or post-MI)

INVESTIGATION
- ECG: conduction defect: BBB
- CXR: pulmonary plethora
- TTE/TOE: site, size, shunt calculation and associated lesions
- Cardiac catheterization: consideration of closure

MANAGEMENT
Surgical (pericardial patch) or percutaneous (Amplatzer® device) closure of haemodynamically significant defects.

ASSOCIATIONS WITH VSD
1. **Fallot's tetralogy**
   - Right ventricular hypertrophy
   - Overriding aorta
   - VSD
   - Pulmonary stenosis

Blalock–Taussig (BT) shunts
- Partially corrects the Fallot's abnormality by anastomosing the subclavian artery to the pulmonary artery
- Absent radial pulse and scar

Other causes of an absent radial pulse
- **Acute:** embolism, aortic dissection, trauma, e.g. radial artery sheath
- **Chronic:** atherosclerosis, coarctation, Takayasu's arteritis ('pulseless disease')

2. **Coarctation**
   A congenital narrowing of the aortic arch that is usually distal to the left subclavian artery.

Clinical signs
- Hypertension in right ± left arm (coarctation usually occurs between left common carotid and left subclavian arteries)
- Prominent upper body pulses, absent/weak femoral pulses, radiofemoral delay
- Heaving pressure loaded apex
- Auscultation: continuous murmur from the coarctation and collaterals radiating through to the back. There is a loud A_2. There may be murmurs from associated lesions

Discussion
ASSOCIATIONS
- **Cardiac:** VSD, bicuspid aortic valve and PDA
- **Non-cardiac:** Turner's syndrome and Berry aneurysms

INVESTIGATION
- ECG: LVH and RBBB
- CXR: rib notching, double aortic knuckle (post-stenotic dilatation)

MANAGEMENT
- Percutaneous: endovascular aortic repair (EVAR)
- Surgical: Dacron patch aortoplasty
- Long-term anti-hypertensive therapy
- Long-term follow-up/surveillance with MRA: late aneurysms and recoarctation

3. **Patent ductus arteriosus (PDA)**
   Continuity between the aorta and pulmonary trunk with left to right shunt
   Risk factor: rubella

Clinical signs
- Collapsing pulse
- Thrill second left inter-space
- Thrusting apex beat
- Auscultation: loud continuous 'machinery murmur' loudest below the left clavicle in systole

Discussion
COMPLICATIONS
- Eisenmenger's syndrome (5%)
- Endocarditis

MANAGEMENT
- Closed surgically or percutaneously

Hypertrophic (obstructive) cardiomyopathy

This young man has complained of palpitations whilst playing football. Examine his cardiovascular system.

Clinical signs

- Jerky pulse character
- Double apical impulse (palpable atrial and ventricular contraction)
- Thrill at the lower left sternal edge
- Auscultation:

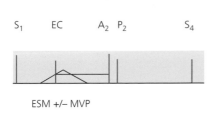

S_1 EC A_2 P_2 S_4

ESM +/– MVP

Ejection systolic murmur (ESM) at the lower left sternal edge that radiates throughout the precordium. A fourth heartsound (S_4) is present due to blood hitting a hypertrophied stiff LV during atrial systole. Dynamic ESM accentuated by reducing LV volume, e.g. standing from squatting or during a strain phase of Valsalva.

- There may be associated mitral valve prolapse (MVP) (see page 52)
- There may be features of Friedreich's ataxia or myotonic dystrophy (see Neurology section)

Discussion

INVESTIGATION

- ECG: LVH with strain (deep T-wave inversion across precordial leads)
- CXR: often normal
- TTE: asymmetrical septal hypertrophy and systolic anterior motion of the anterior mitral leaflet across the LVOT due to misalignment of septal papillary muscle, LVOT gradient (rest/exercise or dobutamine stress)
- Cardiac MR: identifies apical HCM more reliably than TTE
- Cardiac catheterization: gradient accentuated by a ventricular ectopic or pharmacological stress, identification of septals
- Genetic tests: sarcomeric proteins mutation

MANAGEMENT

Asymptomatic:
- Avoidance of strenuous exercise, dehydration and vasodilators

Symptomatic and LVOT gradient >30 mm Hg
- β-Blockers
- Pacemaker
- Alcohol septal ablation
- Surgical myomectomy

Rhythm disturbance/high-risk SCD
- ICD

Refractory:
- Cardiac transplant

Genetic counselling of first-degree relatives (autosomal dominant inheritance)

PROGNOSIS
- Annual mortality rate in adults is 2.5%
- Poor prognosis factors:
  - Young age at diagnosis
  - Syncope
  - Family history of sudden death
  - Septal thickness > 3 cm

Dystrophia myotonica

This man complains of worsening weakness in his hands. Please examine him.

Clinical signs

FACE
- Myopathic facies: long, thin and expressionless
- Wasting of facial muscles and sternocleidomastoid
- Bilateral ptosis
- Frontal balding
- Dysarthria: due to myotonia of tongue and pharynx

HANDS
- **Myotonia:** 'Grip my hand, now let go' (may be obscured by profound weakness). 'Screw up your eyes tightly shut, now open them'.
- **Wasting** and **weakness** of distal muscles with areflexia.
- **Percussion myotonia:** percuss thenar eminence and watch for involuntary thumb flexion.

ADDITIONAL SIGNS
- Cataracts
- Cardiomyopathy, brady- and tachy-arrhythmias (look for pacemaker scar)
- Diabetes (ask to dip urine)
- Testicular atrophy
- Dysphagia (ask about swallowing)

Discussion

GENETICS
- Dystrophia myotonica (DM) can be categorised as type 1 or 2 depending on the underling genetic defect.
  - DM1: expansion of CTG trinucleotide repeat sequence within *DMPK* gene on chromosome 19
  - DM2: expansion of CCTG tetranucleotide repeat sequence within *ZNF9* gene on chromosome 3
- **Genetic anticipation**: worsening severity of the condition and earlier age of presentation within successive generations. Seen in DM1 and also occurs in Huntington's chorea (autosomal dominant) and Friedrich's ataxia (autosomal recessive).
- Both DM1 and 2 are autosomal dominant
- DM1 usually presents in 20s–40s (DM2 later), but can be very variable depending on number of triplet repeats.

DIAGNOSIS
- Clinical features
- EMG: 'dive-bomber' potentials
- Genetic testing

MANAGEMENT
- Affected individuals die prematurely of respiratory and cardiac complications
- Weakness is major problem – no treatment
- Phenytoin may help myotonia
- Advise against general anaesthetic (high risk of respiratory/cardiac complications)

COMMON CAUSES OF PTOSIS

Bilateral	Unilateral
Myotonic dystrophy	Third nerve palsy
Myasthenia gravis	Horner's syndrome
Congenital	

Cerebellar syndrome

This 37-year-old woman has noticed increasing problems with her coordination. Please examine her and suggest a diagnosis.

Clinical signs

Brief conversation   Scanning dysarthria
Outstretched arms   Rebound phenomenon
Movements:
Upper limbs   Finger–nose incoordination   Dysdiadochokinesis
                    Hypotonia   Hyporeflexia
Eyes   Nystagmus
Lower limbs   Heel–shin   Foot tapping
                    Wide-based gait

- Direction of nystagmus: clue to the site of the lesion
- Cerebellar vermis lesions produce an ataxic trunk and gait but the limbs are normal when tested on the bed
- Cerebellar lobe lesions produce **ipsilateral** cerebellar signs in the limbs

Discussion
MNEMONIC FOR SIGNS
Dysdiadochokinesis

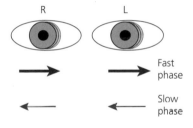

The direction of the fast phase determines the direction of the nystagmus.

Cerebellar lesion
The fast-phase direction is TOWARDS the side of the lesion, and is maximal on looking TOWARDS the lesion.

Vestibular nucleus/VIII nerve lesion
The fast-phase direction is AWAY FROM the side of the lesion, and is maximal on looking AWAY FROM the lesion.

In this case the nystagmus could be due to a cerebellar lesion on the LEFT or a vestibular nucleus lesion on the RIGHT.

Ataxia
Nystagmus
Intention tremor
Scanning dysarthria
Hypotonia/hyporeflexia

AND CAUSES
Paraneoplastic cerebellar syndrome
Alcoholic cerebellar degeneration
Sclerosis (MS)
Tumour (posterior fossa SOL)
Rare (Friedrich's and ataxia telangiectasia)
Iatrogenic (phenytoin toxicity)
Endocrine (hypothyroidism)
Stroke (brain stem vascular event)

AETIOLOGICAL CLUES

• Internuclear opthalmoplegia, spasticity, female, younger age	MS
• Optic atrophy	MS and Friedrich's ataxia
• Clubbing, tar-stained fingers, radiotherapy burn	Bronchial carcinoma
• Stigmata of liver disease, unkempt appearance	EtOH
• Neuropathy	EtOH and Friedrich's ataxia
• Gingival hypertrophy	Phenytoin

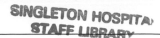
Multiple sclerosis

This 30-year-old woman complains of double vision and incoordination with previous episodes of weakness. Please perform a neurological examination.

Clinical signs

- **Inspection:** ataxic handshake and wheelchair
- **Cranial nerves:** internuclear ophthalmoplegia (frequently bilateral in MS), optic atrophy, reduced visual acuity, and any other cranial nerve palsy

INTERNUCLEAR OPHTHALMOPLEGIA

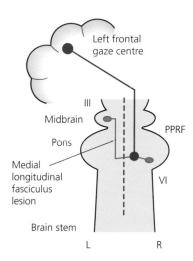

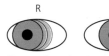

On looking to the right, the right eye abducts normally but the left eye is unable to adduct. The right eye has nystagmus.

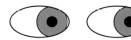

Both eyes look to the left normally.

Both eyes converge normally.

- **Peripheral nervous system:** Upper-motor neurone spasticity, weakness, brisk reflexes and altered sensation
- **Cerebellar:** 'DANISH' (see cerebellar syndrome section)

Discussion

DIAGNOSTIC CRITERIA

Central nervous system demyelination (plaques) causing neurological impairment that is disseminated in both **time** and **space**.

CAUSE

Unknown, but both genetic – (HLA-DR2, interleukin-2 and -7 receptors) and environmental factors (increasing incidence with increasing latitude, association with Epstein–Barr virus infection) appear to play a role.

INVESTIGATION: CLINICAL DIAGNOSIS PLUS

- CSF: oligoclonal IgG bands
- MRI: periventricular white matter plaques
- Visual evoked potentials (VEPs): delayed velocity but normal amplitude (evidence of previous optic neuritis)

OTHER CLINICAL FEATURES
- Higher mental function: depression, occasionally euphoria
- Autonomic: urinary retention/incontinence, impotence and bowel problems
  Uthoff's phenomenon: worsening of symptoms after a hot bath or exercise
  Lhermitte's sign: lightening pains down the spine on neck flexion due to cervical cord plaques

TREATMENT
Multidisciplinary approach
Nurse, physiotherapist, occupational therapist, social worker and physician.

Disease modifying treatments
- Interferon-beta and Glatiramer reduce relapse rate but don't affect progression.
- Monoclonal antibody therapy potentially offers greater benefits; reducing disease progression and accumulated disability, e.g. Alemtuzumab (anti-CD52) – lymphocyte depletion, Natalizumab (anti-α4 integrin) – blocks T-cell trafficking. Toxicity may limit their use.

Symptomatic treatments
- Methyl-prednisolone during the acute phase may shorten the duration of the 'attack' but does not affect the prognosis.
- Anti-spasmodics, e.g. Baclofen.
- Carbamazepine (for neuropathic pain).
- Laxatives and intermittent catheterization/oxybutynin for bowel and bladder disturbance.

PROGNOSIS
Variable: The majority will remain ambulant at 10 years.

MS AND PREGNANCY
- Reduced relapse rate during pregnancy
- Increased risk of relapse in postpartum period
- Safe for foetus (possibly reduced birth weight)

IMPAIRMENT, DISABILITY AND HANDICAP
- Arm paralysis is the impairment
- Inability to write is the disability
- Subsequent inability to work as an accountant is the handicap

Occupational therapy aims to help minimize the disability and abolish the handicap of arm paresis.

Stroke

Examine this patient's limbs neurologically and then proceed to examine anything else that you feel is important.

Clinical signs

- **Inspection:** walking aids, nasogastric tube or PEG tube, posture (flexed upper limbs and extended lower limbs), wasted or oedematous on affected side.
- **Tone:** spastic rigidity, 'clasp knife' (resistance to movement, then sudden release). Ankles may demonstrate clonus (>4 beats).
- **Power:** reduced.

MRC graded:

0, none
1, flicker
2, moves with gravity neutralized
3, moves against gravity
4, reduced power against resistance
5, normal

Extensors are usually weaker than flexors in the upper limbs and vice versa in the lower limbs.

- **Coordination:** sometimes reduced. Usually impaired due to weakness but may reflect cerebellar involvement in posterior circulation stroke.
- **Reflexes:** brisk with extensor plantars

OFFER TO

- Walk the patient if they are able to, to demonstrate the flexed posture of the upper limb and 'tip toeing' of the lower limb.
- Test sensation (this is tricky and should be avoided if possible!). Proprioception is important for rehabilitation.

Other signs

- Upper motor neurone unilateral facial weakness (spares frontalis due to its dual innervation).
- Gag reflex and swallow to minimize aspiration.
- Visual fields and higher cortical functions, e.g. neglect helps determine a Bamford classification.
- **Cause:** irregular pulse (AF), blood pressure, cardiac murmurs or carotid bruits (anterior circulation stroke).

Discussion

DEFINITIONS

- **Stroke:** rapid onset, focal neurological deficit due to a vascular lesion lasting > 24 hours.
- **Transient ischaemic attack (TIA):** focal neurological deficit lasting < 24 hours.

INVESTIGATION

- **Bloods:** FBC, CRP/ESR (young CVA may be due to arteritis), glucose and renal function
- **ECG:** AF or previous infarction
- **CXR:** cardiomegaly or aspiration
- **CT head:** infarct or bleed, territory
- Consider echocardiogram, carotid Doppler, MRI/A/V (dissection or venous sinus thrombosis in young patient), clotting screen (thrombophilia), vasulitis screen in young CVA

Management

ACUTE
- Thrombolysis with tPA (within 4.5 hours of acute ischaemic stroke)
- Clopidogrel (or aspirin + dipyridamole)
- Referral to a specialist stroke unit: **multidisciplinary approach:** physiotherapy, occupational therapy, speech and language therapy and specialist stroke rehabilitation nurses
- DVT prophylaxis

CHRONIC
- Carotid endarterectomy in patients who have made a good recovery, e.g. in PACS (if >70% stenosis of the ipsilateral internal carotid artery)
- Anticoagulation for cardiac thromboembolism
- Address cardiovascular risk factors
- Nursing +/− social care.

BAMFORD CLASSIFICATION OF STROKE (LANCET 1991)
Total anterior circulation stroke (TACS)
- **H**emiplegia (contra-lateral to the lesion)
- **H**omonomous hemianopia (contra-lateral to the lesion)
- **H**igher cortical dysfunction, e.g. dysphasia, dyspraxia and neglect

Partial anterior circulation (PACS)
- 2/3 of the above

Lacunar (LACS)
- Pure hemi-motor or sensory loss

Prognosis at 1 year (%)

	TACS	PACS	LACS
Dead	60	15	10
Dependent	35	30	30
Independent	5	55	60

DOMINANT PARIETAL-LOBE CORTICAL SIGNS
- **Dysphasia:** receptive, expressive or global
- **Gerstmann's syndrome**
  - Dysgraphia, dyslexia and dyscalculia
  - L-R disorientation
  - Finger agnosia

NON-DOMINANT PARIETAL-LOBE SIGNS
- Dressing and constructional apraxia
- Spatial neglect

EITHER
- Sensory and visual inattention
- Astereognosis
- Graphaesthesia

VISUAL FIELD DEFECTS

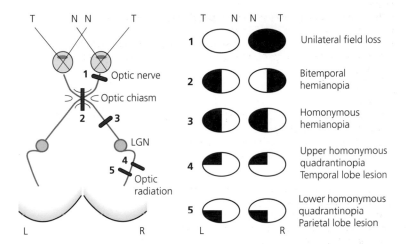

Lateral medullary (Wallenberg) syndrome

- Most common brainstem vascular syndrome
- Due to occlusion of posterior inferior cerebellar artery (PICA)
- Often variable in its presentation

BRAINSTEM STRUCTURES AFFECTED BY RIGHT-SIDED LESION

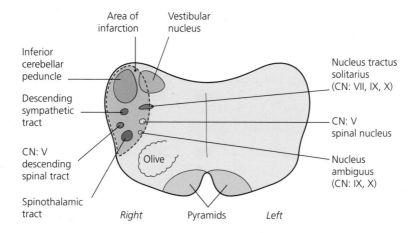

CLINICAL CONSEQUENCES OF THIS LESION

Localisation	Clinical sign(s)	Brainstem structure affected
Ipsilateral to lesion (e.g. on right with right-sided infarction)	Cerebellar signs	Inferior cerebellar peduncle
	Nystagmus (Present with vertigo and vomiting)	Vestibular nucleus
	Horner syndrome	Descending sympathetic tract
	Palatal paralysis and decreased gag reflex	Nucleus ambiguus (CN IX and X)
	Loss of trigeminal pain and temperature sensation	Trigeminal nerve (CN V) spinal nucleus and tract
Contralateral to lesion (e.g. on left with right-sided lesion)	Loss of pain and temperature sensation	Spinothalamic tract

Spastic legs

Examine this man's lower limbs neurologically. He has had difficulty in walking.

Clinical signs

- Wheelchair and walking sticks (disuse atrophy and contractures may be present if chronic)
- Increased tone and ankle clonus
- Generalized weakness
- Hyper-reflexia and extensor plantars
- Gait: 'scissoring'

ADDITIONAL SIGNS

- Examine for a sensory level suggestive of a spinal lesion
- Look at the back for scars or spinal deformity
- Search for features of multiple sclerosis, e.g. cerebellar signs, fundoscopy for optic atrophy
- Ask about bladder symptoms and note the presence or absence of urinary catheter. Offer to test anal tone

Discussion

COMMON CAUSES

- Multiple sclerosis
- Spinal cord compression/cervical myelopathy
- Trauma
- Motor neurone disease (no sensory signs)

OTHER CAUSES

- Anterior spinal artery thrombosis: dissociated sensory loss with preservation of dorsal columns
- Syringomyelia: with typical upper limb signs
- Hereditary spastic paraplegia: stiffness exceeds weakness, positive family history
- Subacute combined degeneration of the cord: absent reflexes with upgoing plantars
- Friedreich's ataxia
- Parasagittal falx meningioma

CORD COMPRESSION

- **Medical emergency**
- **Causes:**
  - **Disc prolapse** (above L1/2)
  - Malignancy
  - Infection: abscess or TB
  - Trauma: # vertebra
- **Investigation of choice:** spinal MRI
- **Treatment:**
  - Urgent surgical decompression
  - Consider steroids and radiotherapy (for a malignant cause)

LUMBO-SACRAL ROOT LEVELS

L 2/3	Hip flexion	
L 3/4	Knee extension	**Knee jerk L 3/4**
L 4/5	Foot dorsi-flexion	
L 5/S 1	Knee flexion	
	Hip extension	
S 1/2	Foot plantar-flexion	**Ankle jerk S 1/2**

LOWER LIMB DERMATOMES

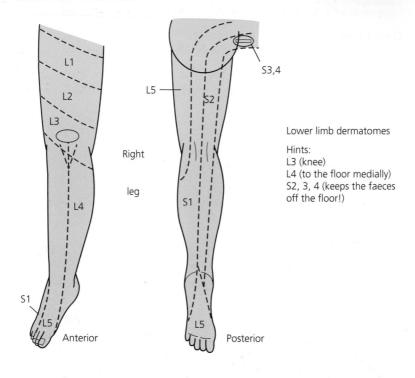

Lower limb dermatomes

Hints:
L3 (knee)
L4 (to the floor medially)
S2, 3, 4 (keeps the faeces off the floor!)

Syringomyelia

Examine this patient's upper limbs neurologically. He has been complaining of numb hands.

Clinical signs

- Weakness and wasting of small muscles of the hand
- Loss of reflexes in the upper limbs
- Dissociated sensory loss in upper limbs and chest: loss of pain and temperature sensation (spinothalamic) with preservation of joint position and vibration sense (dorsal columns)
- Scars from painless burns
- Charcot joints: elbow and shoulder

Additional signs

- Pyramidal weakness in lower limbs with upgoing (extensor) plantars
- Kyphoscoliosis is common
- Horner's syndrome (see Ophthalmology section)
- If syrinx extends into brain stem (syringobulbia) there may be cerebellar and lower cranial nerve signs

Discussion

- Syringomyelia is caused by a progressively expanding fluid filled cavity (syrinx) within the cervical cord, typically spanning several levels.

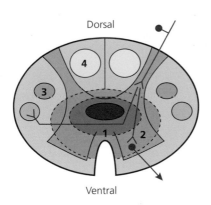

Dorsal

Ventral

Syrinx expands ventrally affecting:

1 Decussating spinothalamic neurones producing segmental pain and temperature loss at the level of the syrinx.

2 Anterior horn cells producing segmental lower motor neurone weakness at the level of the syrinx.

3 Corticospinal tract producing upper motor neurone weakness below the level of the syrinx.

It usually spares the dorsal columns 4 (proprioception).

- The signs may be asymmetrical.
- Frequently associated with an Arnold–Chiari malformation and spina bifida.
- Investigation = spinal MRI.

CHARCOT JOINT (NEUROPATHIC ARTHROPATHY)

- Painless deformity and destruction of a joint with new bone formation following repeated minor trauma secondary to loss of pain sensation.
- The most important causes are:
  - Tabes dorsalis: hip and knee
  - Diabetes: foot and ankle
  - Syringomyelia: elbow and shoulder
- Treatment: bisphosphonates can help

CERVICAL ROOTS

C 5/6	Elbow flexion and supination	**Biceps and supinator jerks C 5/6**
C 7/8	Elbow extension	**Triceps jerk C 7/8**
T 1	Finger adduction	

UPPER LIMB DERMATOMES

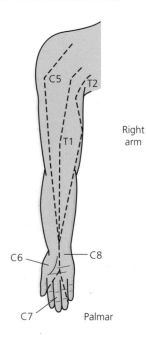

Right arm

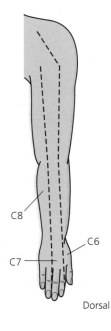

Palmar

Dorsal

Upper limb dermatomes

Hints:
C6 thumb
C7 middle finger
C8 little finger

Motor neurone disease

This man complains of gradually increasing weakness. Please examine him neurologically.

Clinical signs
- **Inspection:** wasting and fasciculation
- **Tone:** usually spastic but can be flaccid
- **Power:** weak
- **Reflexes:** absent and/or brisk. (Absent knee jerk with extensor plantar reflexes.)
- **Sensory examination is normal**
- **Speech:** dysarthria may be bulbar (nasal, 'Donald Duck' speech, due to palatal weakness) or pseudo-bulbar ('hot potato' speech, due to a spastic tongue).
- **Tongue:** wasting and fasciculation (bulbar) or a stiff spastic tongue with brisk jaw jerk (pseudo-bulbar).
- There is no sensory, extra-ocular muscle, cerebellar or extra-pyramidal involvement. Sphincter and cognitive disturbance occasionally seen.

Discussion
- MND is a progressive disease of unknown aetiology
- There is axonal degeneration of upper and lower motor neurones

Motor neurone disease may be classified into three types, although there is often some overlap:

- **Amyotrophic lateral sclerosis** (50%): affecting the cortico-spinal tracts predominantly producing **spastic** paraparesis or tetraparesis.
- **Progressive muscular atrophy** (25%): affecting anterior horn cells predominantly producing wasting, fasciculation and weakness. **Best prognosis**.
- **Progressive bulbar palsy** (25%): affecting lower cranial nerves and suprabulbar nuclei producing speech and swallow problems. **Worst prognosis**.

INVESTIGATION
- Clinical diagnosis
- **EMG:** fasciculation
- **MRI (brain and spine):** excludes the main differential diagnoses of cervical cord compression and myelopathy and brain stem lesions

TREATMENT
- Supportive, e.g. PEG feeding and NIPPV
- Multidisciplinary approach to care
- Riluzole (glutamate antagonist): slows disease progression by an average of 3 months but does not improve function or quality of life and is costly

PROGNOSIS
- Most die within 3 years of diagnosis from bronchopneumonia and respiratory failure. Some disease variants may survive longer.
- Worst if elderly at onset, female and with bulbar involvement.

CAUSES OF GENERALIZED WASTING OF HAND MUSCLES
- **Anterior horn cell**
  - MND
  - Syringomyelia
  - Cervical cord compression
  - Polio

- **Brachial plexus**
  - Cervical rib
  - Pancoast's tumour
  - Trauma
- **Peripheral nerve**
  - Combined median and ulnar nerve lesions
  - Peripheral neuropathy
- **Muscle**
  - Disuse atrophy, e.g. rheumatoid arthritis

FASCICULATION
- Visible muscle twitching at rest
- Cause: axonal loss results in the surviving axons recruiting and innervating more myofibrils than usual resulting in large motor units
- Seen commonly in MND and syringomyelia

Parkinson's disease
This man complains of a persistent tremor. Examine him neurologically.

Clinical signs
- Expressionless face with an absence of spontaneous movements.
- Coarse, pill-rolling, 3–5 Hz tremor. Characteristically asymmetrical.
- **Bradykinesia** (demonstrated by asking patient to repeatedly oppose each digit onto thumb in quick succession).
- **Cogwheel rigidity** at wrists (enhanced by synkinesis – simultaneous movement of the other limb (tap opposite hand on knee, or wave arm up and down)).
- Gait is shuffling and festinant. Absence of arm swinging – often asymmetrical.
- Speech is slow, faint and monotonous.

In addition
- **BP** looking for evidence of **multisystem atrophy:** Parkinsonism with postural hypotension, cerebellar and pyramidal signs.
- Test **vertical eye movements** (up and down) for evidence of **progressive supranuclear palsy**.
- **Dementia** and Parkinsonism: **Lewy-body dementia**.
- Ask for a **medication** history.

Discussion
CAUSES OF PARKINSONISM
Parkinson's disease (idiopathic)
Parkinson plus syndromes:
    Multisystem atrophy (Shy–Drager)
    Progressive supranuclear palsy (Steele–Richardson–Olszewski)
    Corticobasal degeneration; unilateral Parkinsonian signs
Drug-induced, particularly phenothiazines
Anoxic brain damage
Post-encephalitis
MPTP toxicity ('frozen addict syndrome')

PATHOLOGY
- Degeneration of the dopaminergic neurones between the substantia nigra and basal ganglia.

TREATMENT
- **L-Dopa** with a peripheral Dopa-decarboxylase inhibitor, e.g. Madopar/co-beneldopa:
  - Problems with nausea and dyskinesia
  - Effects wear off after a few years so generally delay treatment as long as possible
  - End-of-dose effect and on/off motor fluctuation may be reduced by modified release preparations
- **Dopamine agonists**, e.g. Pergolide:
  - Use in younger patients: less side effects (nausea and hallucinations) and save L-Dopa until necessary
  - **Apomorpine** (also dopamine agonist) given as an SC injection or infusion; rescue therapy for patients with severe 'off' periods
- **MAO-B inhibitor**, e.g. Selegiline, inhibit the breakdown of dopamine
- **Anti-cholinergics**, can reduce tremor, particularly drug-induced
- **COMT inhibitors**, e.g. Entacapone, inhibit peripheral breakdown of L-Dopa thus reducing motor fluctuations
- **Amantadine**, increases dopamine release
- Surgery; deep-brain stimulation (to either the subthalamic nucleus or globus pallidus) helps symptoms

CAUSES OF TREMOR
- **Resting tremor:** Parkinson's disease
- **Postural tremor** (worse with arms outstretched):
  - Benign essential tremor (50% familial) improves with EtOH
  - Anxiety
  - Thyrotoxicosis
  - Metabolic: CO_2 and hepatic encephalopathy
  - Alcohol
- **Intention tremor:** seen in cerebellar disease

Hereditary sensory motor neuropathy

This man complains of progressive weakness and a change in the appearance of his legs. Please examine him neurologically.

Clinical signs
- Wasting of distal lower limb muscles with preservation of the thigh muscle bulk (inverted champagne bottle appearance)
- Pes cavus (seen also in Friedreich's ataxia)
- Weakness of ankle dorsi-flexion and toe extension
- Variable degree of stocking distribution sensory loss (usually mild)
- Gait is high stepping (due to foot drop) and stamping (absent proprioception)
- Wasting of hand muscles
- Palpable lateral popliteal nerve

Discussion
- The commonest HSMN types are I (demyelinating) and II (axonal).
- Autosomal dominant inheritance (test for PMP22 mutations in HSMN I).
- HSMN is also known as Charcot–Marie–Tooth disease and peroneal muscular atrophy.

OTHER CAUSES OF PERIPHERAL NEUROPATHY
Predominantly sensory
- Diabetes mellitus
- Alcohol
- Drugs, e.g. isoniazid and vincristine
- Vitamin deficiency, e.g. B_{12} and B_1

Predominantly motor
- Guillain–Barré and botulism present acutely
- Lead toxicity
- Porphyria
- HSMN

Mononeuritis multiplex
- Diabetes mellitus
- Connective tissue disease, e.g. SLE and rheumatoid arthritis
- Vasculitis, e.g. polyarteritis nodosa and Churg–Strauss
- Infection, e.g. HIV
- Malignancy

Friedreich's ataxia
Examine this young man's neurological system.

Clinical signs
- Young adult, wheelchair (or ataxic gait)
- Pes cavus
- Bilateral cerebellar ataxia (ataxic hand shake + other arm signs, dysarthria, nystagmus)
- Leg wasting with absent reflexes and bilateral upgoing plantars
- Posterior column signs (loss of vibration and joint position sense)

Other signs
- Kyphoscoliosis
- Optic atrophy (30%)
- High-arched palate
- Sensorineural deafness (10%)
- Listen for murmur of HOCM
- Ask to dip urine (10% develop diabetes)

Discussion
- Inheritance is usually autosomal recessive
- Onset is during teenage years
- Survival rarely exceeds 20 years from diagnosis
- There is an association with HOCM and a mild dementia

CAUSES OF EXTENSOR PLANTARS WITH ABSENT KNEE JERKS
- Friedreich's ataxia
- Subacute combined degeneration of the cord
- Motor neurone disease
- Taboparesis
- Conus medullaris lesions
- Combined upper and lower pathology, e.g. cervical spondylosis with peripheral neuropathy

Facial nerve palsy

Examine this patient's cranial nerves. What is wrong?

Clinical signs

- Unilateral facial droop, absent nasolabial fold and forehead creases
- Inability to raise the eyebrows (frontalis), screw the eyes up (orbicularis oculi) or smile (orbicularis oris)

Bell's phenomenon: eyeball rolls upwards on attempted eye closure.

LEVEL OF THE LESION

- **Pons**   +VI palsy and long tract signs
  - MS and stroke
- **Cerebellar-pontine angle**   +V, VI, VIII and cerebellar signs
  - Tumour, e.g. acoustic neuroma
- **Auditory/facial canal**   +VIII
  - Cholesteatoma and abscess
- **Neck and face**   + scars or parotid mass
  - Tumour and trauma

Discussion

COMMONEST CAUSE IS BELL'S PALSY

- Rapid onset (1–2 days)
- HSV-1 has been implicated
- Induced swelling and compression of the nerve within the facial canal causes demyelination and temporary conduction block
- Treatment: prednisolone commenced within 72 hours of onset improves outcomes, plus aciclovir if severe
- **Remember eye protection** (artificial tears, tape eye closed at night)
- Prognosis: 70–80% make a full recovery; substantial minority have persistent facial weakness
- Pregnancy: Bell's palsy is more common in pregnancy, and outcome may be worse

OTHER CAUSES OF A VII NERVE PALSY

- Herpes zoster (Ramsay–Hunt syndrome)
- Mononeuropathy due to diabetes, sarcoidosis or Lyme disease
- Tumour/trauma
- MS/stroke

CAUSES OF BILATERAL FACIAL PALSY

- Guillain–Barré   • Myasthenia gravis
- Sarcoidosis   • Bilateral Bell's palsy
- Lyme disease

Myasthenia gravis

Examine this patient's cranial nerves. She has been suffering with double vision.

Clinical signs
- Bilateral ptosis (worse on sustained upward gaze)
- Complicated bilateral extra-ocular muscle palsies
- Myasthenic snarl (on attempting to smile)
- Nasal speech, palatal weakness and poor swallow (bulbar involvement)
- Demonstrate proximal muscle weakness in the upper limbs and **fatiguability**. The reflexes are normal
- Look for sternotomy scars (thymectomy)
- State that you would like to assess respiratory muscle function (FVC)

Discussion
- **Associations:** other autoimmune diseases, e.g. diabetes mellitus, rheumatoid arthritis, thyrotoxicosis, SLE and thymomas
- **Cause:** Anti-nicotinic acetylcholine receptor (anti-AChR) antibodies affect motor end-plate neurotransmission

INVESTIGATIONS
Diagnostic tests
- Anti-AChR antibodies positive in 90% of cases
- Anti-MuSK (muscle-specific kinase) antibodies often positive if anti-AChR negative
- EMG: decremented response to a titanic train of impulses
- Edrophonium (Tensilon) test: an acetylcholine esterase inhibitor increases the concentration of ACh at the motor end plate and hence improves the muscle weakness. **Can cause heart block and even asystole**.

OTHER TESTS
- CT or MRI of the mediastinum (thymoma in 10%)
- TFTs (Grave's present in 5%)

TREATMENTS
Acute
- IV immunoglobulin or plasmapheresis (if severe)

Chronic
- Acetylcholine esterase inhibitor, e.g. pyridostigmine
- Immunosuppression: steroids and azathioprine
- Thymectomy is beneficial even if the patient does not have a thymoma (usually young females)

Lambert–Eaton myasthenic syndrome (LEMS)
- Diminished reflexes that become brisker after exercise
- Lower limb girdle weakness (unlike myasthenia gravis)
- Associated with malignancy, e.g. small-cell lung cancer
- Antibodies block pre-synaptic calcium channels
- EMG shows a 'second wind' phenomenon on repetitive stimulation

CAUSES OF BILATERAL EXTRA-OCULAR PALSIES
- Myasthenia gravis
- Graves' disease
- Mitochondrial cytopathies, e.g. Kearns–Sayre syndrome

- Miller–Fisher variant of Guillain–Barré syndrome
- Cavernous sinus pathology

CAUSES OF BILATERAL PTOSIS
- Congenital
- Senile
- Myasthenia gravis
- Myotonic dystrophy
- Mitochondrial cytopathies, e.g. Kearns–Sayre syndrome
- Bilateral Horner's syndrome

Tuberous sclerosis

This patient has had a first seizure recently. Please examine them as you wish. What is the diagnosis?

Clinical signs

SKIN CHANGES
- Facial (perinasal: butterfly distribution) adenoma sebaceum (angiofibromata)
- Periungual fibromas (hands and feet)
- Shagreen patch: roughened, leathery skin over the lumbar region
- Ash leaf macules: depigmented macules on trunk (fluoresce with UV/Wood's light)

RESPIRATORY
- Cystic lung disease

ABDOMINAL
- Renal enlargement caused by polycystic kidneys and/or renal angiomyolipomata
- Transplanted kidney
- Dialysis fistulae

EYES
- Retinal phakomas (dense white patches) in 50%

CNS
- Mental retardation may occur
- Seizures
- Signs of anti-epileptic treatment, e.g. phenytoin: gum hypertrophy and hirsuitism

Discussion
- Autosomal dominant (*TSC1* on chromosome 9, *TSC2* on chromosome 16) with variable penetrance
- 80% have epilepsy (majority present in childhood; but adult presentation also seen)
- Cognitive defects in 50%

RENAL MANIFESTATIONS
- Include renal angiomyolipomas, renal cysts and renal cell carcinoma
- The genes for tuberous sclerosis and ADPKD are contiguous on chromosome 16, hence some mutations lead to both conditions
- Renal failure may result from cystic disease, or parenchymal destruction by massive angiomyolipomas

INVESTIGATION
- Skull films: 'railroad track' calcification
- CT/MRI head: tuberous masses in cerebral cortex (often calcify)
- Echo and abdominal ultrasound: hamartomas and renal cysts

Previously known as **EPILOIA** (**EPI**lepsy, **LO**w **I**ntelligence, **A**denoma sebaceum)

Neurofibromatosis
Examine this patient's skin.

Clinical signs
- Cutaneous neurofibromas: two or more
- Café au lait patches: six or more, >15 mm diameter in adults
- Axillary freckling
- Lisch nodules: melanocytic hamartomas of the iris
- Blood pressure: hypertension (associated with renal artery stenosis and phaeochromocytoma)
- Examine the chest: fine crackles (honeycomb lung and fibrosis)
- Neuropathy with enlarged palpable nerves
- Visual acuity: optic glioma/compression

Discussion
- Inheritance is autosomal dominant
- Type I (chromosome 17) is the classical peripheral form
- Type II (chromosome 22) is central and presents with bilateral acoustic neuromas and sensi-neural deafness rather than skin lesions

ASSOCIATIONS
- Phaeochromocytoma (2%)
- Renal artery stenosis (2%)

COMPLICATIONS
- Epilepsy
- Sarcomatous change (5%)
- Scoliosis (5%)
- Mental retardation (10%)

CAUSES OF ENLARGED NERVES AND PERIPHERAL NEUROPATHY
- **Neurofibromatosis**
- Leprosy
- Amyloidosis
- Acromegaly
- Refsum's disease

Abnormal pupils

Examine this patient's eyes.

Horner's pupil
Clinical signs

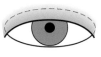

Horner's

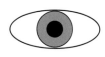

'PEAS'
Ptosis (levator palpebrae is
partially supplied by sympathetic
fibres)
Enophthalmos (sunken eye)
Anhydrosis (sympathetic fibres
control sweating)
Small pupil (miosis)

May also have flushed/warm skin
ipsilaterally to the Horner's pupil
due to loss of vasomotor
sympathetic tone to the face.

Extra points
• Look at the ipsilateral side of the neck for scars (trauma, e.g. central lines, carotid
endarterectomy surgery or aneurysms) and tumours (Pancoast's).

Discussion
CAUSE
Following the sympathetic tract's anatomical course:

Brain stem	Spinal cord	Neck
MS	Syrinx	Aneurysm
Stroke (Wallenberg's)		Trauma Pancoast's

Holmes–Adie (myotonic) pupil
Clinical signs

Holmes–Adie pupil

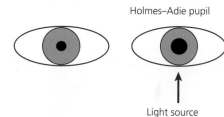

Light source

Moderately dilated pupil that
has a poor response to light
and a sluggish response
to accommodation
(you may have to wait!)

Extra points
• Absent or diminished ankle and knee jerks

Discussion
A benign condition that is more common in females. Reassure the patient that nothing is
wrong.

Argyll Robertson pupil
Clinical signs

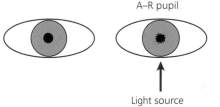

A–R pupil

Small irregular pupil
Accommodates but doesn't
   react to light
Atrophied and depigmented iris

Light source

Extra points
• Offer to look for sensory ataxia (tabes dorsalis)

Discussion
• Usually a manifestation of quaternary syphilis, but it may also be caused by diabetes mellitus
• Test for quaternary syphilis using TPHA or FTA, which remain positive for the duration of the illness
• Treat with penicillin

Oculomotor (III) nerve palsy
Clinical signs

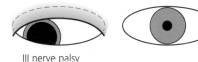

III nerve palsy

Ptosis usually complete
Dilated pupil
The eye points 'down and out' due
to the unopposed action of lateral
rectus (VI) and superior oblique (IV)

Extra points

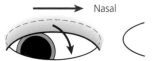

Nasal

Test for the trochlear (IV) nerve
On looking nasally the eye will intort (rotate
towards the nose) indicating that the trochlear
nerve is working

• If the pupil is normal consider medical causes of III palsy
• Surgical causes often impinge on the superficially located papillary fibres running in the III nerve

Discussion
CAUSES

Medical	Surgical
Mononeuritis multiplex, e.g. DM	Communicating artery aneurysm (posterior)
Midbrain infarction: Weber's Midbrain demyelination (MS)	Cavernous sinus pathology: thrombosis, tumour or fistula (IV, V and VI may also be affected)
Migraine	Cerebral uncus herniation

Optic atrophy
Examine this woman's eyes.

Clinical signs
- Relative afferent pupillary defect (RAPD): dilatation of the pupil on moving the light source from the normal eye (consensual reflex) to the abnormal eye (direct reflex):

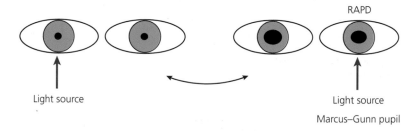

RAPD

Light source   Light source

Marcus–Gunn pupil

- Fundoscopy: disc pallor

Extra points
Look for the cause.

ON EXAMINING THE FUNDUS
- **Glaucoma** (cupping of the disc)
- **Retinitis pigmentosa**
- **Central retinal artery occlusion**
- **Frontal brain tumour: Foster–Kennedy syndrome** (papilloedema in one eye due to raised intercranial pressure and optic atrophy in the other due to direct compression by the tumour)

AT A GLANCE FROM THE END OF THE BED
- Cerebellar signs, e.g. nystagmus: **multiple sclerosis** (internuclear ophthalmoplegia), **Friedreich's ataxia** (scoliosis and pes cavus)
- Large bossed skull: **Paget's disease** (hearing aid)
- Argyll–Robertson pupil: **Tertiary syphilis**

Discussion
CAUSES: PALE DISCS
PRESSURE*: tumour, glaucoma and Paget's
ATAXIA: Friedreich's ataxia
LEBER'S
DIETARY: ↓B$_{12}$, **D**EGENERATIVE: retinitis pigmentosa
ISCHAEMIA: central retinal artery occlusion
SYPHILIS and other infections, e.g. CMV and toxoplasmosis
CYANIDE and other toxins, e.g. alcohol, lead and tobacco
SCLEROSIS*: MS
(* denotes commonest cause)

RETINAL PATHOLOGY

These cases may appear in isolation as part of the Neurology Station, or within Station 5 (e.g. retinal artery occlusion and AF). Other retinal pathology is covered elsewhere (e.g. diabetic retinopathy in Station 5).

Age-related macular degeneration (AMD)

Examine this elderly patient's fundi. She complains of recent loss of vision.

Clinical signs

- Wet (neovascular and exudative) or dry (non-neovascular, atrophic and non-exudative)
- Macular changes:
  - ○ Drusen (extracellular material)
  - ○ Geographic atrophy
  - ○ Fibrosis
  - ○ Neovascularization (wet)

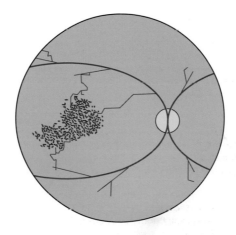

Discussion

RISK FACTORS

- Age, white race, family history and smoking
- Wet AMD have a higher incidence of coronary heart disease and stroke

TREATMENT

- Ophthalmology referral
- Wet AMD may be treated by intravitreal injections of anti-VEGF (though can increase cerebrovascular and cardiovascular risk)

PROGNOSIS

- Majority of patients progress to blindness in the affected eye within 2 years of diagnosis

Retinitis pigmentosa

This man has been complaining of difficulty seeing at night. Please examine his eyes.

Clinical signs
- White stick and braille book (registered blind)
- Reduced peripheral field of vision (tunnel vision)
- Fundoscopy

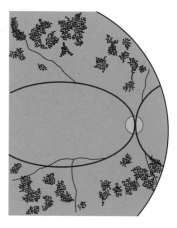

Peripheral retina 'bone spicule pigmentation', which follows the veins and spares the macula.

Optic atrophy due to neuronal loss (consecutive).

Association: cataract (absent red reflex).

'At a glance' findings can help make the diagnosis:

- **Ataxic:** Friedreich's ataxia, abetalipoproteinaemia, Refsum's disease, Kearns–Sayre syndrome
- **Deafness (hearing-aid/white stick with red stripes):** Refsum's disease, Kearns–Sayre syndrome, Usher's disease
- **Ophthalmoplegia/ptosis and permanent pacemaker:** Kearns–Sayre syndrome
- **Polydactyly:** Laurence–Moon–Biedl syndrome
- **Icthyosis:** Refsum's disease

Discussion
- Inherited form of retinal degeneration characterized by loss of photo receptors

CAUSES
- Congenital: often autosomal recessive inheritance, 15% due to rhodopsin pigment mutations
- Acquired: post-inflammatory retinitis

PROGNOSIS
- Progressive loss of vision due to retinal degeneration. Begins with reduced night vision. Most are registered blind at 40 years, with central visual loss in the seventh decade
- No treatment although vitamin A may slow disease progression

CAUSES OF TUNNEL VISION
- Papilloedema
- Glaucoma
- Choroidoretinitis
- Migraine
- Hysteria

Retinal artery occlusion

Examine this man's fundi.

Clinical signs
- Pale, milky fundus with thread-like arterioles
- ± Cherry red macula (choroidal blood supply)
- **Cause:** AF (irregular pulse) or carotid stenosis (bruit)
- **Effect:** optic atrophy and blind (white stick)

Note that branch retinal artery occlusion will have a field defect opposite to the quadrant of affected retina

Discussion
CAUSES
- **Embolic:** carotid plaque rupture or cardiac mural thrombus
  Treatment: aspirin, anti-coagulation and endarterectomy
- **Giant cell arteritis:** tender scalp and pulseless temporal arteries
  Treatment: high-dose steroid urgently, check ESR and arrange temporal artery biopsy to confirm diagnosis

Retinal vein occlusion

Examine this patient's fundi.

Clinical signs

- Flame haemorrhages +++ radiating out from a swollen disc
- Engorged tortuous veins
- Cotton wool spots
- **Cause:** look for diabetic or hypertensive changes (visible in branch retinal vein occlusion).
- **Effect:** Rubeosis iridis causes secondary glaucoma (in central retinal vein occlusion), visual loss or field defect.

Discussion

CAUSES

- **Hypertension**
- **Hyperglycaemia:** diabetes mellitus
- **Hyperviscocity:** Waldenström's macroglobulinaemia or myeloma
- **High intraocular pressure:** glaucoma

Station 4
Ethics, Law and
Communication Skills

Clinical mark sheet

Clinical skill	Satisfactory	Unsatisfactory
Clinical Communication Skills	Relevant, accurate, clear, structured, comprehensive, fluent, professional	Omits important information inaccurate, unclear, unstructured, uses jargon, unpractised
Managing Patients' Concerns	Seeks, detects & addresses concerns Listens, confirms understanding, empathetic	Over-looks concerns Poor listening, not empathetic Does not check patient understanding
Clinical Judgement	Sensible and appropriate management plan, applies clinical/ legal/ ethical knowledge appropriately	Inappropriate management Does not apply clinical, legal or ethical knowledge to the case
Maintaining Patient Welfare	Respectful, sensitive Ensures comfort, safety and dignity	Causes physical or emotional discomfort Jeopardises patient safety

Cases for PACES, Third Edition. Stephen Hoole, Andrew Fry and Rachel Davies.
© 2015 John Wiley & Sons, Ltd. Published 2015 by John Wiley & Sons, Ltd.

ETHICS AND LAW IN MEDICINE

Principles of medical ethics

Most ethical dilemmas can be resolved, at least in part, by considering the four cornerstones of any ethical argument, namely **autonomy, beneficence, non-maleficence** and **justice**.

- **Autonomy** 'self-rule': respecting and following the patient's decisions in the management of their condition.
- **Beneficence:** promoting what is in the patient's best interests.
- **Non-maleficence:** avoiding harm.
- **Justice:** doing what is good for the population as a whole. Distributing resources fairly.

There is often not a right or wrong answer to tricky ethical problems but this framework enables informed discussion.

EXAMPLE
- PEG feeding a semi-conscious patient post-CVA:
  Autonomy: the patient wishes to be fed, or not.
  Beneficence and **non-maleficence:** feeding may improve nutritional status and aid recovery, but with risks of complication from the insertion of the PEG tube and subsequent aspiration. Also, the patient's poor quality of life may be lengthened.
  Justice: heavy resource burden looking after PEG-fed patients in nursing homes.

Medico-legal system

The legal system of England and Wales (Scottish legal system is different) is defined by **Common (Case) Law** and **Statute (Acts of Parliament) Law** and may be subdivided into **Public (Criminal) Law** and **Private (Civil) Law**. Court decisions follow **judicial precedent** – they follow judgements that have gone before.

Medical malpractice is commonly a breach of the **Law of Tort** (part of Civil Law) and the most important of these are **negligence** and **battery** (a part of the tort of trespass). The judge must decide, on the balance of probabilities (rather than beyond reasonable doubt – Criminal law) whether the defendant(s) (doctor and hospital NHS Trust) are liable and whether the Claimant is due compensation.

Negligence

This is the commonest reason for a doctor to go to court. Claimants need to prove:

1. The doctor had a duty of care:
   - Doctors (unless they are GPs in their geographical practice) are not legally obliged to act as 'Good Samaratans' (although morally they may be)
2. There was a breach of the appropriate standard of care:
   - The Bolam test: the doctor is not negligent if he or she acted in accordance with a responsible/reasonable/respectable body of medical opinion (even if that opinion is in the minority)
   - The Bolitho test: the opinion must also withstand logical analysis
3. The breach of the duty of care caused harm

Competency and consent

A competent patient

Every human being of adult years and of sound mind has a right to determine what shall be done to his or her own body.

In accepting a patient's autonomy to determine the course of management the clinician must be satisfied that the patient has capacity. If this is not the case, the doctor should act in the patient's best interests.

Consent is only valid when the individual has capacity (or in legal terms, 'is competent').

- A patient is not incompetent because they act against their best interests.
- Capacity is not a global term but is specific to each decision, i.e. a patient may be competent to make a will but at the same time incompetent to consent to treatment.
- A clinician does not have to prove beyond all reasonable doubt that a patient has capacity, only that the balance of probability favours capacity.

Assessing capacity

In order to be assessed as having capacity to make a specific decision, a patient must be able to:

1. Comprehend and retain the information needed
2. Be able to understand the pros and cons of both accepting and refusing the proposed plan
3. Be free from undue external influence
4. Be able to communicate his or her response. Patient must be free from external influence
   - Patients under 16 years of age can consent to undergo, but not refuse treatment if they are deemed '**Gillick competent**', i.e. are deemed mature enough to understand the implications of their actions. However, refusal of consent to treatment may be overridden by a parent or a court, if it is in the child's best interest.

Legal aspects

- **Assault** is a threat or an attempt to physically injure another, whereas **battery** is actual (direct or indirect) physical contact or injury without consent. They are usually civil rather criminal offenses.
- **Implied consent:** if a patient goes to hospital and holds out their arm to allow a medical practitioner to take their pulse – written or verbal consent is not necessary.
- **Consent documentation:** If a patient does not receive certain relevant information when consented for a procedure a doctor may be found negligent. It is advisable to tell the patient of all potential serious complications and those with an incidence of at least 1%. A signed consent form is not legally binding – patients may withdraw consent at any time. It is not illegal to operate without a consent form (as long as verbal or implied consent has been obtained). However, it provides admissible evidence that consent has been obtained.
- It is best practice to discuss any intended procedure with a relative and their agreement documented on the consent form if the patient lacks capacity, but this is not legally binding and does not constitute consent.

The Mental Capacity Act (2005)

The Mental Capacity Act was introduced to protect people who cannot make decisions for themselves. It enables people to appoint someone on their behalf in case they become unable to make decisions for themselves in the future. There are three parts to this act which you need to be aware of and please note that this is a separate act from the Mental Health Act:

1. Appointment of a Deputy
   An individual can nominate a Deputy to make decisions with regards to monetary matters. An individual needs to be legally competent when this application is made and the application needs to be accepted by the Court of Protection to be valid. The Deputy must make decisions in accordance with the best interests of the individual. A Deputy does not have the right to make decisions about medical or welfare issues on behalf of the individual.
2. Appointment of a Lasting Power of Attorney
   An Attorney appointed through a Lasting Power of Attorney application has two roles: firstly to act on behalf of an individual with regards to monetary and property matters, but also, in the event of a person losing capacity to make medical or welfare decisions, an Attorney can act as a patient proxy; that is, the opinion of the Attorney needs to be taken into account as if it were the opinion of the patient themselves. An application has to be signed by a solicitor and then registered with the Office of the Public Guardian. There is a separate form for each role and different individuals can be appointed for each task. The Attorney must act in the best interests of the individual and abide by the Code of Practice. If anyone disputes the decision of an Attorney, particularly if they are refusing life-saving treatment, the Court of Protection ultimately adjudicates on the decision. Just as with a patient, an Attorney cannot demand treatment that is deemed to be clinically inappropriate.
3. Independent Mental Capacity Advocate
   When a person loses capacity and has not previously appointed a Deputy or Attorney, the Public Guardian, through the Court of Protection, can appoint an independent person to help with welfare and monetary decisions. They will liaise with doctors, nurses and social workers to agree a decision in the best interests of the patient.

ASSESSING THE BEST INTERESTS OF A PATIENT
When making a decision about the treatment of patient who has lost capacity one needs to take into account the following points:

1. the patient's wishes or beliefs as well as those carers or relatives of the patient
2. the circumstances of the decision and whether the patient may regain capacity in the future to allow them to make the decision
3. whether or not the decision about life saving therapy is motivated by the thought to bring about death.

ADVANCED DECISIONS TO REFUSE TREATMENT
Advanced decisions to refuse treatment (ADRT), previously known as Advanced Directives, can be written by a person who has capacity and who wishes to express decisions to refuse treatment in the future, should they lose the ability to express their wishes or they lose capacity to make decisions. The ADRT can be verbally expressed to a third party but it is best if it is a written document signed by a witness. This witness does not need to be a solicitor or other professional and can be a family member. It is recommended that the document contains the name and address of the individual expressing their wishes, the name and address of their GP, that the document is dated, that the wishes of the individual are clearly documented including the circumstances in which the decision would apply and if the decision is to refuse a life-saving or life-sustaining treatment, such as antibiotics for pneumonia, that the phrase 'even if life is at risk' is documented. A copy should be forwarded to the individual's GP. A doctor can be at risk of battery if he/she does not comply with the wishes expressed in a ADRT document. The doctor needs to be satisfied

that the individual had capacity at the time of the writing of the document, that they were free of coercion at that time and that they fully understood the consequences of their wishes.

The Mental Health Act
The Mental Health Act 1983 can only be evoked to treat psychiatric illness in non-consenting patients.

Section 5(2): emergency doctor's holding power
- Applied by a physician of any speciality on an *in-patient* to enable a psychiatric assessment to be made
- 72 hours duration
- Good practice to convert this to a Section 2 or 3

Section 2: admission for assessment order
- Applied by two written medical recommendations (usually a psychiatrist and a GP) and an approved social worker or relative, on a patient *in the community*
- 28 days duration
- May be converted to a Section 3
- The patient has a right of appeal to a tribunal within 14 days of detention

Section 3: admission for treatment order
- Applied as in a Section 2 on a patient already diagnosed with a mental disorder
- 6 months duration then reviewed

Section 4: emergency admission to hospital order
- Applied by one doctor (usually a GP) and an approved social worker or relative
- Urgent necessity is demonstrable
- May be converted to a Section 2 or 3

Confidentiality

Confidentiality is an implied contract necessary for a successful doctor-patient relationship. Without it, a patient's autonomy and privacy is compromised, trust is lost and the relationship weakened.

GMC Guidelines (*Confidentiality: Protecting and Providing Information*, September 2000, Section 1 – Patients' right to confidentiality, Paragraph 1)

> Patients have the right to expect that doctors will not disclose any personal information which they learn during the course of their professional duties, unless the patient gives specific permission (preferably in writing). Without assurances about confidentiality patients may be reluctant to give doctors the information they need to provide good care.

Legal aspects

- Patients usually complain to the GMC rather than sue if there has been a breach of confidentiality.
- Under common law doctors are legally obliged to maintain confidentiality although this obligation is not absolute.
- Maintenance of confidentiality is a public not a private interest – it is in the public's interest to be able to trust a doctor. Therefore, breaching confidentiality is a question of balancing public interests.
- Doctors have **discretion** to breach confidentiality when another party may be at serious risk of harm, e.g. an epileptic who continues to drive (the GMC advises doctors to inform the DVLA medical officer) or an HIV-positive patient who refuses to tell their sexual partner. They may also share information within the medical team.
- Doctors **must** breach confidentiality to the relevant authorities in the following situations:
  - Notifiable diseases
  - Drug addiction
  - Abortion
  - In vitro fertilization
  - Organ transplant
  - Births and deaths
  - Police request
  - Search warrant signed by a circuit judge
  - Court order
  - Prevention, apprehension or prosecution of terrorists or perpetrators of serious crime

How to do it

No breach of confidentiality has occurred if a patient gives consent or the patient cannot be identified. If consent is not given to disclose information but a physician deems that a breach in confidentiality is necessary, the patient should be notified in writing of the reason for disclosure, the content, to whom the disclosure has been made and the likely consequence for the patient.

The GMC provides guidelines on when confidentiality may be breached, which do not have the force of the law but are taken seriously by the courts. These guidelines may be consulted at: www.gmc-uk.org.

End of life decisions
This is a contentious area and medical opinion is diverse.

Sanctity of life
The view that whenever possible human life should be maintained, could be argued as ethically unjustified if extending that life results in suffering (non-maleficence) and if trivial life extension occurs at enormous monetary expense (justice).

Killing versus letting die
In the former, the doctor actively causes the patient's death, in the latter the patient's illness causes death, i.e. 'nature takes its course' whilst the doctor is passive. However, some disagree stating the decision to act or to omit to act are both 'active' choices, which may make it more difficult to morally justify.

Withholding versus withdrawing treatment
Although it may be easier to withhold treatment, rather than to withdraw that which has been started already, there are no legal or necessarily moral distinctions between the two. Withdrawing treatment is considered in law to be a passive act and not killing.

EXAMPLE
A hospital trust was granted permission from the House of Lords to discontinue artificial hydration and nutrition in a young patient in a persistent vegetative state (Airedale NHS Trust v Bland, 1993). This case established the equivalence of withholding and withdrawing care and that the basic provisions of food and water are classified as medical treatments that could be withdrawn.

Doctrine of double effect
This is a moral argument that distinguishes actions that are intended to harm versus those where harm is foreseen but not intended.

EXAMPLE
The administration of morphine intended to palliate pain in a patient with a terminal illness may have the foreseen consequence of respiratory arrest and subsequent death. It is morally and legally acceptable though because the primary aim was to alleviate pain, not cause death.

Do-not-attempt cardio-pulmonary resuscitation (DNA-CPR) orders
In 2014, a case was brought to the UK Court of Appeal (Tracey v Cambridgeshire NHS Foundation Hospitals Trust) by a family questioning whether or not it was against Article 8 of the Human Rights Act not to discuss DNA-CPR orders with a patient or their family. The judge ruled in favour of Tracey and it is therefore now a legal obligation for medical staff to consult a patient or, in the situation where a patient lacks capacity, their family or advocate, when a decision to withhold potentially life-saving treatment is being considered, including DNA-CPR. Failure to discuss these decisions could potentially result in legal action and it is no longer acceptable to avoid these discussions on the grounds that they may cause undue distress to the patient or family.

It is important to realise that this ruling does not state that CPR must be offered to all patients, it is merely stating that the decision whether or not to perform CPR must be discussed with the patient. English law still states that doctors are not required to administer futile treatments and this can include CPR.

Euthanasia
Euthanasia is intentional killing, i.e. murder under English law and therefore illegal. Assisted suicide, i.e. helping someone take their own life, is also a criminal offence.

ARGUMENTS FOR
- Respecting a patient's autonomy over their body
- Beneficence, i.e. 'mercy killing', may prevent suffering
- Suicide is legal but is unavailable to the disabled

ARGUMENTS AGAINST
- Good palliative care obviates the need for euthanasia
- Risk of manipulation/coercion/exploitation of the vulnerable
- Undesirable practices will occur when constraints on killing are loosened ('**slippery-slope' argument**)

Communication skills
Breaking bad news
If done well this can help the patient come to terms with their illness and minimize psychological distress. There are no hard and fast rules, but a patient-centred approach often helps.

How to do it
- Choose a setting that is private and free from disturbance (give your bleep to someone else). Have enough time to do it properly.
- Invite other health care workers, e.g. a nurse, for support and to ensure continuity of information given by all the team.
- Introduce yourself and the purpose of the discussion.
- Offer the opportunity for relatives to attend if the patient wishes. This is useful for patient support and can help the dissemination of information.
- Check the patient's existing awareness and gauge how much they want to be told.
- Give the bad news clearly and simply. Avoid medical jargon. Avoid information overload. Avoid 'loose terminology' that may be misinterpreted.
- Pause and acknowledge distress. Wait for the patient to guide the conversation and explore their concerns as they arise.
- If you are unsure as to exact treatment options available, inform the patient that their case is going to be discussed at an MDT (be it cancer or other disease group) and a decision made at that meeting as to best care. Arrange to meet them immediately after this meeting.
- Recap what has been discussed and check understanding.
- Bring the discussion to a close but offer an opportunity to speak again and elicit the help of other groups, e.g. specialist cancer nurses or societies, to help the patient at this difficult time.
- Enquire how the patient is planning on getting home. If distressed, advise them that they should not drive. Offer to ring a relative to collect them or to arrange a taxi home.

Other problems
- **Denial:** If a patient is in denial reiterate the key message that needs to be addressed. Confront the inconsistencies in their perceptions and if this does not work, acknowledge their denial in a sensitive way. It may be better to leave this to a later date, perhaps when the patient is ready to confront the painful reality.
- **Anger:** This is a natural and usually transient part of the grieving process. 'Shooting the messenger' can occur occasionally, particularly if the news is delivered poorly. Acknowledge their anger and empathize with their plight. If this does not diffuse the situation, terminate the session and reconvene later.
- **'How long have I got?':** Explore why the patient wants to know. Answer in broad terms: hours–days, days–weeks, etc.

Points for the exam
Use real days of the week for the MDT and a date for the follow-up appointment: 'We have our meeting at 8 am on Wednesday morning. I will contact you after this and then see you in the clinic on Thursday 10 June at 3 pm.'

Dealing with a difficult patient
How to do it
AN ANGRY PATIENT
- Listen without interruption and let them voice their anger
- Keep calm and do not raise your voice
- Acknowledge they are angry and try to explore why
- Empathize by stating that you understand why they are upset but try to avoid saying that you 'know how they feel'
- Apologize if there has been an error
- Volunteer that if they wish to take matters further that they could contact the Patient Advice and Liason Service or give them information about the trust's complaints procedure. Most trusts have a leaflet with this information on it.

A NON-COMPLIANT PATIENT
- Explore why they have not taken their medication. Were the side effects bothering them? Was the drug not working?
- Educate the patient. Perhaps they were not aware how important it was to take the tablets.
- Offer solutions. Direct supervision of treatment, e.g. anti-tuberculosis treatment. Offer to change the therapy if possible.

A SELF-DISCHARGING PATIENT
- Explain why you do not want them to leave.
- If they have capacity they may leave but do so at their own risk and against medical advice. To attempt to stop them is assault.
- If they lack capacity to make this decision they can be detained by reasonable force, acting in their best interests under common law. To let them go is negligent. However, if in attempting to detain such a person there is risk of serious injury to the patient or those restraining the patient, then you may have no alternative but to let them go. If you are presented with this scenario, in the discussion make it clear to the examiners that you would phone the GP and also attempt to contact relatives of the patient to inform them of the events and that the patient might be at risk.
- Patients with smear positive TB (AFBs present in sputum and therefore posing a risk of infection to the public) can be detained, but not treated, under the Public Health Act.

A PATIENT THAT CONTINUES TO DRIVE DESPITE CONTRAINDICATION
Although it is the duty of the patient (not the doctor) to declare a disability that precludes him or her from holding a UK driving licence, it is one of the acknowledged circumstances (stated by the GMC) under which a breach of confidentiality may be justified.

- Try and persuade the patient to inform the DVLA. Mention lack of insurance cover if they drive and safety issues to themselves and other road users. They can also face a £1000 fine if they do not inform the DVLA of a listed medical condition.
- Ask them to provide written evidence that they have informed the DVLA if you suspect they have not.
- Inform the patient that you will write to the DVLA if they fail to do so.
- Write to the DVLA if no evidence is forthcoming and to the patient to inform them you have done so.

Driving restrictions

Disease	Private vehicle licence	HGV/PSV licence
First unprovoked seizure with a low rate of recurrence	6 months if fit free/medical review	5 years if risk of recurrence is <2% per annum
	6 months during treatment changes	
Epilepsy (2 or more seizures)	1 year if fit free/medical review	10 years if fit free off medication
ACS	**1 month** if untreated	**6 weeks** if symptom free and no inducible ischaemia on ETT
	1 week if treated with stent and normal LV	
Stroke/TIA	**1 month** if no persistent deficit	**1 year** if no persistent deficit
IDDM	**Notify DVLA** may drive if no visual impairment and aware of hypoglycaemia	**Banned**

Any illness where the doctor feels that the patient's ability to drive is significantly impaired should be referred to the DVLA for further action and the patient is told not to drive in the mean time.

Other issues to address
- Explore the impact on the patient's job and lifestyle.
- How is the patient going to get home from your clinic?
  For full guidelines: http://www.dvla.gov.uk/medical/ataglance.aspx

Information delivery

Communication skills are frequently assessed by the candidate's ability to inform the patient about their medical condition. These scenarios are frequently executed poorly by candidates in the PACES examination. Make sure that you conduct a structured interview and that you have time to cover all relevant points. Candidates often underestimate how difficult it is do to these scenarios well. Think about what you might say in a given scenario in advance of the exam.

How to do it

- Introduce yourself and establish the reason for the discussion.
- Assess the patient's level of knowledge. Firstly, discuss the nature of the condition that they have been diagnosed with. Give the information in simple language avoiding medical jargon. Rehearse prior to the examination a description of all common medical complaints.
- Facilitate questions and answer them, but avoid digressing too much.
- Next discuss the medication they are going home on. Make sure that you fully explain the indications for and how to use any PRN medication, particularly when to use a GTN spray or salbutamol inhaler. Discuss any important side effects, particularly if you need the patient to report any adverse events, e.g. jaundice while on TB therapy.
- Try to ascertain if anything precipitated this admission, e.g. recent acquisition of a long-haired cat in the household of a patient presenting with acute asthma.
- Address any lifestyle issues which may be negatively impacting on the condition, e.g. smoking, weight, high alcohol use.
- Formulate a plan of action with the patient.
- Reiterate your discussion with the patient to ensure understanding.
- Offer further information sources, e.g. leaflets, societies or groups.
- Organize appropriate follow-up.
- Close the interview.

Tips

- Read the case scenario carefully and structure your interview in 5 minutes beforehand. Jot down the headings and take them into the room as an aide memoire: Explanation of condition; Discussion of regular and PRN medications; Side effects; Lifestyle; Follow-Up; Leaflets.
- This is a role-play station so use your imagination.
- If you are asked a question by the patient and you do not know the answer, say that you are unable to answer at present but you will find out next time (as you would in real life!).
- Be aware of possible legal and ethical facets to the case and pre-empt the examiners by tackling them in the case before the discussion.
- Body language speaks volumes.

Worked examples
Epilepsy

An 18-year-old woman who is trying to become a professional model has had her second grand mal seizure in 3 months, which was witnessed by her GP. She has had a normal CT head and metabolic causes have been excluded. She has returned to your outpatient clinic for the results. Please discuss the diagnosis with her.

- The diagnosis is epilepsy. Explain what this means to the patient in lay terms: *disorganized electrical activity in the brain* **(see 'Information delivery' section).**
- Explore **social aspects:**
  - She has been drinking a lot of alcohol recently and staying out late at all night parties.
  - She drives to modelling agencies and relies heavily on her car.
  - She hates taking tablets.
- Discuss **treatment** options to limit her seizure activity:
  - Avoid excess alcohol and sleep deprivation.
  - Avoid precipitants, e.g. flashing disco lights.
    Drugs: there are some newer anti-epileptic medications, e.g. lamotrigine, that have fewer side effects. This is important to her as she is a model!
- Stress **compliance (if poor compliance see 'Dealing with a difficult patient' section):**
  - It is imperative that if she is on the oral contraceptive combined pill, she is told the risks of **pill failure**. This is important, as anti-epileptics are teratogenic. Advise alternative forms of contraception, e.g. barrier or if this is unacceptable switch to a higher dose oestrogen pill or progesterone pill.
  - If she wants to become **pregnant,** it is a balance of risk between a seizure when pregnant, which carries a significant risk of miscarriage and the potential teratogenic side effects of the drugs. Most physicians encourage female patients wishing to start a family to continue on their epileptic treatment. Remember folate supplements!
    Safety issues
  - Avoid swimming or bathing alone and heights.
  - Driving restrictions **(if she continues to drive see 'Dealing with a difficult patient' and 'Breaking confidentiality' sections).**
- **Recap** the important points and formulate an agreed plan.
- **Check understanding** and answer her questions.
- **Other information:** offer leaflets, British Epilepsy Society (www.epilepsy.org.uk), contact numbers and an appointment with epilepsy specialist nurse.
- Conclude the interview after ascertaining how she is going to get home.

Huntington's chorea

A 26-year-old son of your patient has requested to see you, to discuss his mother's diagnosis. She has developed a dementing illness and chorea in her late forties. Her father committed suicide at the age of 60. A diagnosis of Huntington's chorea has been made on genetic testing. She currently lives in her own home but is not coping. She has also asked her son to help her die. Discuss the relevant issues with her son. He is 'trying for a family'.

- Ascertain that his mother has consented to this discussion to avoid the **confidentiality** pitfall, and a rather short interview!
  Remember if the mother is your patient and the son is not, you only have a duty of care to the mother. If she does not want you to discuss the diagnosis with her son, then to do so would breach confidentiality.

- Explain Huntington's chorea and its inheritance to the son **(see 'Information delivery' and 'Breaking bad news' sections)**. Emphasize that there is **no cure** and management is supportive.
- How the diagnosis **relates to him** and his family.
  Anticipation, i.e. if he is affected the onset may be at an earlier age.
  Genetic screening and family planning. Prenatal screening. This would potentially result in an abortion – briefly explore this with the patient.
- Life insurance and employment implications.
- How the diagnosis **relates to his mother**.
  Social aspects: community care or nursing home placement plans.
  Legal aspects: advanced decisions to refuse treatment (previously known as advanced directives), lasting power of attorney may be discussed **(see 'Consent and competency' section)**.
  Assisted suicide is illegal **(see 'End of life decisions' section)**.
- **Recap** and formulate an agreed plan.
- **Check understanding** and answer questions.
- **Other information:** offer leaflets, Huntington's society contact numbers and an appointment with a geneticist. An appointment with a social worker would be useful to organize residential care for his mother.
- **Arrange follow-up** ideally with all the family as it affects all of them.
- Conclude the interview.

Tips for the exam

This is a complex question and a candidate could lose marks by not covering all the points raised in the scenario. Make notes in the 5 minutes before you go into the station with headings to include: Consent; Explanation of Huntington's disease; Care of the mother; Impact of diagnosis on son, his future children and any other family members; How to manage the request to help her die. Watch the clock as one could easily spend the allotted time just covering the genetic aspects of this scenario.

Paracetamol overdose

A patient arrives in the emergency medical unit having taken 50 paracetamol tablets 4 hours ago. She says she wants to die and does not want to be treated although she would like painkillers for her abdominal pain. Negotiate a treatment plan with this patient.

POINTS TO DISCUSS
- Be clear on the amount of paracetamol taken and the time of ingestion as this will influence the management, i.e. calculating the treatment level of paracetamol.
- Alcoholism or anti-epileptic medication lowers the treatment line.
- Assess the suicidal intent, e.g. letter.
- Previous psychiatric history.
- Negotiate an agreed **treatment plan** if possible.
- Organize a referral to the deliberate self-harm team.
- **Recap** and **check understanding**.
- Conclude the interview.

TREATMENT DEBATE
- **Competency:**
  - Does she understand that this overdose is life-threatening and what the treatment involves?
  - Is the paracetamol overdose affecting her judgment?
  - Is a psychiatric illness affecting her judgment, e.g. delusional?
- If deemed to lack capacity then you must act in her best interests and treat her against her will under **common law**.
- If she has capacity she has a right to refuse treatment.

If you do not treat and the patient dies, you may have to defend this decision in court. If you treat her in the face of her wishes, you could be charged with battery. Most courts will not find physicians that act in the patient's best interests guilty.

- **Implied consent:** May be invoked to defend treatment of a patient that arrives in hospital having taken an overdose but they may have been taken there against their will, or they may have attended hospital to palliate their symptoms.
- **Advanced decision to refuse treatment** Notes stating they do not wish to be treated may be ignored, because the attending physician often cannot be sure of the circumstances in which it was written, e.g. under duress, or that the patient has not changed her mind.
- **The Mental Health Act** cannot be invoked to treat overdose patients, even if they have depression.
- Attempted suicide is no longer illegal in the UK. Assisting someone to commit suicide is illegal.

If in doubt it is prudent to treat overdose patients under common law, acting in their best interests. It may be advisable to seek legal advice.

Brain stem death and organ donation
You are working in intensive care and you have recently admitted a 30-year-old man who was hit by a car. He has sustained a severe head injury and his second assessment of brain stem function show he is brain stem dead. You have found an organ donor card in his wallet. Please discuss the diagnosis with his mother and father and broach the subject of organ donation with them.

POINTS TO DISCUSS
Brain stem death

- Explain that he has had a severe brain injury and that he is brain dead **(see 'Breaking bad news' section)**.
- **Inform them about brain death**.
- 'He has **died** and only the ventilator is keeping his other organs working'.
- Pause for reflection and questions.

Organ donation

- Broach in a sensitive way: 'I know this is a very difficult time for you both but did you know that your son carried a donor card?'
- Points that can be addressed may include:
  - The need for **an operation** to 'harvest' the organs.
  - **HIV testing** prior to donation.
  - Not all the organs taken may be used.
  - Time delays involved prior to the certification of death and the release of the body.
- Avoid information overload and be guided by the relative's questions and the time available.
- Offer to put them in touch with the **transplant coordinator** for the region. They will be able to counsel them further.
- Remind them that a decision has to be made swiftly but avoid harassing the relatives unduly (offer to come back when they have had a chance to think about it).

Being too involved in the transplantation program may be ethically wrong for an ITU physician, due to potentially conflicting interests.

A donor card is sufficient legal authority to proceed (advanced directive although the signature is not witnessed). However, it is good practice to assess the relatives' wishes and few centres would proceed if the relatives did not assent to organ donation.

- **Recap** and formulate a plan.
- **Check understanding** at each stage and answer their questions.
- **Offer other information:** leaflet on transplantation.
- Conclude the interview.

Tip for the exam:
Completing this scenario well hinges on whether you are able to explain to the family about brain death. This is best approached as if you are breaking news that the patient has died. It avoids ambiguity as to whether or not there is any chance of recovery.

BRAIN STEM DEATH AND ORGAN DONATION
As in this case, discussion with a coroner must occur prior to organ donation if it is a coroner's case. Permission may be withheld if a death is due to a criminal action.

HUMAN TISSUE ACT (1961) AND HUMAN ORGAN TRANSPLANT ACT (1989)
Statute law defining codes of practice on organ retrieval, consent and diagnostic tests of brain death.
    To establish brain stem death two consultants assess independently that:

- The cause of death is known and all potentially treatable causes for the patient's state have been excluded, e.g. hypothermia, biochemical derangement and drugs, i.e. the unconscious state is **irreversible** and **permanent**.
- The brain stem reflexes, e.g. pupil, corneal, motor cranial nerve responses, vestibulo-ocular, gag and cough reflexes are absent and there is no spontaneous respiratory drive at a $PaCO_2 > 50\,mm\,Hg$.

All organs are usually harvested with minimum warm ischaemic time, i.e. with a beating heart up to the moment of harvesting (except corneas); hence, these difficult discussions need to be addressed early.

- Contraindications: infections, e.g. HIV and prion disease; metastatic tumours; severe atherosclerosis.
- Be aware of the introduction of 'non-heart beating organ donation'. For further information see GMC guidelines at www.gmc-uk.org.

Non-compliant diabetic
An 18-year-old female insulin-dependent diabetic has been admitted with yet another ketoacidotic episode. She has family problems. You notice she is very thin and has lanugo hair on her face. Please counsel her regarding her poor diabetic control and weight loss.

POINTS TO DISCUSS
- **Diabetic education:**
  - Review insulin regimen, injection sites and **compliance** (may be non-compliant due to weight gain or family problems).
  - Educate about the importance of tight glycaemic control and the dangers of diabetic ketoacidosis.
  - Ask about other cardiovascular risk factors, e.g. smoking.
- **Dieting and anorexia nervosa:**
  - Emphasize the importance of a balanced diet and diabetic control.
  - Explore her dietary intake.

- Ask her about her weight, body image and self-esteem.
- Assess for **depression** (associated with anorexia).
- **Family problems:**
  - Explore these and counsel. Patients suffering from anorexia often have problems at home.
    Family therapy can be useful in treating anorexia nervosa.
- **Recap** and formulate a plan.
- **Check understanding** and answer questions.
- **Offer other information:** leaflets and Anorexia Nervosa Society.
- Conclude the interview.

LEGAL ISSUES
- Capacity: due to the effects of malnutrition on cognition, an anorexic patient may not be competent to refuse treatment.
- Anorexia nervosa can be treated under the **Mental Health Act (1983)** as an outpatient or in severe cases on a specialist unit.
- Food is deemed a treatment for a mental illness and can be given against the patient's will under the Mental Health Act.

Sample questions
Information delivery

- This 60-year-old man is about to leave hospital, 7 days after an uncomplicated MI. He has some concerns regarding his return to normal life. What advice would you give him regarding his condition?
- A 23-year-old newly-diagnosed asthmatic has been recently discharged from hospital and arrives in your outpatient clinic for a review of his illness. He works as a veterinary nurse and smokes 15 cigarettes per day. Educate him about his illness, arrange further tests and instigate a treatment plan.
- A 32-year-old woman has been recently diagnosed with multiple sclerosis following a second episode of optic neuritis. Discuss her diagnosis, prognosis and likely treatment options.
- A 29-year-old man with a 14-year history of ulcerative colitis treated with steroids and ciclosporin has come to your follow-up clinic. He is concerned with some of the side effects he has been having on his medication. Address this and counsel him in the further management of his condition.
- A 50-year-old heavy smoker presents with his fifth exacerbation of COPD this year. He tells you he does not take his inhalers because he thinks they make him worse. His blood gas on air reads a PaO_2 of 6.8. Discuss treatment options with him.

Communicating medico-legal and ethical principles

- A patient with metastatic breast carcinoma attends your clinic. She has read on the Internet that there is a new treatment that might be helpful. Unfortunately, your trust has decided not to fund this treatment at present. Counsel her on these matters.
- A patient's relatives arrive to be told that their father was unfortunately 'dead-on-arrival' to hospital. It is likely he suffered a large myocardial infarction. Break this bad news to them and guide them with regard to the need for a coroner's post-mortem. For religious reasons they would like the body released today.
- A 90-year-old woman who has recently had a debilitating stroke is classified as 'do not attempt resuscitation'. Her daughter has found out that this decision has been made without her consent and demands that her mother be for resuscitation. Discuss the management of this patient with the daughter.
- A patient with motor neurone disease who is now wheelchair-bound has come to your clinic. She believes she is a burden to her family and wants your advice regarding the best way to end her own life. Please counsel her.
- A 24-year-old doctor has come to your clinic. She has recently been on elective to Africa where she sustained a needle stick injury. Initial tests show she is hepatitis C positive. She is reluctant to stop working. Please counsel her.

Station 5
Brief Clinical Consultations

Clinical mark sheet

Clinical skill	Satisfactory	Unsatisfactory
Clinical communication skills	Relevant, focused, fluent, professional	Omits important history Unpractised, unprofessional
Physical examination	Correct, appropriate, practised, professional	Incorrect technique Unfocused, hesitant
Clinical judgement	Sensible and appropriate management	Inappropriate management
Managing patients' concerns	Addresses concerns, listens, empathetic	Over-looks concerns Poor listening Not empathetic
Identifying physical signs	Identifies correct signs Does not find signs that are not present	Misses important signs Finds signs that are not present
Differential diagnosis	Constructs sensible differential diagnosis	Poor differential, fails to consider the correct diagnosis
Maintaining patient welfare	Respectful, sensitive Ensures comfort, safety and dignity	Causes physical or emotional discomfort Jeopardises patient safety

Cases for PACES, Third Edition. Stephen Hoole, Andrew Fry and Rachel Davies.
© 2015 John Wiley & Sons, Ltd. Published 2015 by John Wiley & Sons, Ltd.

This station is designed to bring everything together. It assesses the approach of the candidate to clinical scenarios that will be encounted on take or in a general medical clinic. It lends itself to cases that are multisystemic and have an multidisciplinary focus. Subspecialty cases that do not feature in other stations (e.g. skin, locomotor and endocrine cases) can appear here.

This station is often the hardest to master. Examiners are looking to pass candidates who are not fazed by complexity and who can focus on the key important features of a case. Responding to the clues as they emerge and thinking on your feet is encouraged. Passing this station will demonstrate efficient and effective practice that is required to cope with a busy acute medical take or over-running out-patient clinic. Spending time in these departments will help you prepare.

You have one 5-minute block of preparation time before this station when you will be given the 'statement' for each case. Use this preparatory time wisely: list a few key features of the history and examination that you plan to elicit during the cases, and think about potential differential diagnoses.

You have 8 minutes to assess the patient and discuss your findings with them, and then 2 minutes to present your findings to the examiners and discuss your differential diagnosis. It is imperative that history and examination are performed as both carry marks. There is not much time but do not forget the basics: introduce yourself, be empathetic and maintain patient welfare. These are also assessed. It may be appropriate to examine the patient early in the consultation whilst continuing to take a history. This saves precious time and enables you to help focus your questioning on the problem if the diagnosis is uncertain. But also be flexible and direct your attention to clues as the case unfolds.

Considering the social impact of the disease on the patient is important. To get you started, pulse and BP assessment can be justified in most cases and is a reasonable 'ice-breaker' for any examination.

Cases encountered in this section fall into two broad categories: general presentations (e.g. chest pain, dyspnoea) and specific conditions, often multisystem disorders (e.g. the patient with obvious systemic sclerosis). For the general presentations we suggest the key diagnosis likely to be the focus of the case. For all the cases we list crucial points from the history, important examination findings and discussion topics that may be encountered. This approach is a guide; you may decide that other aspects of the cases deserve more attention. Whatever your focus, be flexible on the day, and prepared to justify your approach to the examiners!

Chest pain

This 54-year-old male smoker has chest pain.

Diagnosis: myocardial ischaemia
Differential diagnosis: pleuritic (PE or pneumonia), musculoskeletal, oeosophageal reflux/spasm

History

ESTABLISH SYMPTOM IS ANGINA
- Character: dull ache, band-like and tightness
- Position/radiation: substernal into arm/jaw
- Exacerbating and relieving factors:
  - ↑ Heavy meals, cold, exertion and emotional stress
  - ↓ Rest and/or sublingual GTN (although may relieve oesophageal spasm as well)
- Associated symptoms: nausea, sweating and breathlessness
- Differential diagnosis: Pleuritic chest pain or cough (lung), history of peptic ulcers (GI), recent heavy lifting (musculoskeletal)

RISK FACTORS FOR CAD
- Smoking, diabetes, family history, cholesterol, ↑BP, age and ethnic origin (South Asian)

IMPACT OF SYMPTOMS ON PROFESSION
- DVLA restrictions

TREATMENT CONSIDERATIONS
- Any contraindications to antiplatelet agents/anticoagulants/thrombolysis
- PVD: femoral pulse for angiography
- Varicose veins: surgical conduits for grafting

Examination

HANDS AND PULSE
- Tar-stained fingers (smoking), pulse rate and rhythm

EYES
- Xanthelasma (cholesterol)

AUSCULTATION
- Heart: murmurs: AS or MR
- Chest bibasal crackles: CCF

PERIPHERIES
- Swollen ankles: CCF

Discussion

INITIAL INVESTIGATIONS
- Acute: 12-lead ECG and CXR, troponin, FBC, creatinine (eGFR), fasting lipid profile and glucose

EMERGENCY TREATMENT
- Antithrombotic/antiplatelet; GpIIb/IIIa inhibitor if high risk (TIMI risk score ≥4)
- Antianginal: GTN and β-blocker
- Risk modifiers: statin and ACE inhibitors
- Coronary angiography (if troponin positive):
  - Angioplasty and stent
  - Surgery: CABG

- Further investigations (if troponin negative):
  - Functional tests to confirm ischaemia: exercise stress test, MIBI scan and stress echo or MRI

TIMI risk score

	Point
Age > 65	1
> 3 risk factors	1
Known CAD	1
Taking aspirin on admission	1
Severe angina (refractory to medication)	1
Troponin elevation	1
ST depression >1 mm	1
> 3 points = high mortality risk	

Headache

This university student has a headache and skin rash.

Diagnosis: bacterial meningitis (most important to exclude)
Differential diagnosis: subarachnoid haemorrhage and migraine

History

SYMPTOMS CONSISTENT WITH MENINGITIS
- **Meningism**: neck stiffness, headache and photophobia
- Nausea and vomiting
- Focal neurological deficit, constitutional symptoms of infection, rash

RISK FACTORS FOR HEADACHE
- Meningitis: immunosuppressed, close meningitis contact and foreign travel
- Subarachnoid haemorrhage: hypertension
- Migraine: triggers, e.g. stress, tiredness, chocolate and red wine

DIFFERENTIAL DIAGNOSIS
- Subarachnoid haemorrhage: sudden onset, severe 'thunderclap' headache, may be preceded by 'warning' sentinel headaches
- Migraine: The mnemonic **POUND**ing headache (**P**ulsating, duration of 4–72 h**O**urs, **U**nilateral, **N**ausea, **D**isabling). May have aura, e.g. scintillating scotoma or focal neurological deficits in 30%

TREATMENT CONSIDERATIONS
- Allergies to penicillin

Examination

LOOK FOR MENINGISM
- Neck stiffness
- Photophobia on fundoscopy
- Kernig's sign: hip flexion and knee: flexion → extension is painful and resisted (avoid causing pain in the exam!)
- Fever

LOOK FOR A RASH
- Meningococcal meningitis: petechial/purpura rash indicates associated septicaemia (does not blanche on compressing)

BRIEF NEUROLOGICAL EXAMINATION
- Cerebral abscess:
  - Localizing signs: upper limb: pronator drift; lower limb: extensor plantar; cranial nerve palsy
- Cerebral oedema/increasing intracranial pressure:
  - Reduced Glasgow Coma Score, unilateral dilated pupil (third nerve palsy) and papilloedema

HAEMODYNAMIC STABILITY
- Septic shock: pulse and BP

Discussion

INVESTIGATION
- Blood culture
- Lumbar puncture:
  - Will need head CT to exclude raised intracranial pressure if localizing signs or altered conscious state

- Send CSF sample for MC + S, glucose (with blood glucose) and protein:
  - Bacterial: low glucose, high protein, neutrophils and gram + cocci
  - Viral: normal glucose and protein, mononuclear cells
- Differentiate bloody tap from subarachnoid haemorrhage by assessing xanthochromia (bilirubin from degraded RBCs turn CSF yellow)

TREATMENT
- Do not delay antibiotics:
  - Penicillin: high dose, intravenous immediately if diagnosis is suspected
- Meningitis is a notifiable disease:
  - Treat close contacts

Swollen calf

This 34 year-old woman has a swollen right leg. Her only medication is the OCP.

Diagnosis: deep vein thrombosis
Differential diagnosis: ruptured Baker's cyst and cellulitis

History

SYMPTOMS OF DVT
- Unilateral swollen and tender calf

RISK FACTORS OF DVT
- Medical conditions, e.g. active cancer or heart failure (prothrombotic states)
- Immobility, e.g. flight, surgery (especially orthopaedic), stroke etc.
- Previous personal or family history of DVT or PE
- Oral contraceptive use in women

DIFFERENTIAL DIAGNOSIS
- Previous knee trauma or joint problem

COMPLICATIONS
- PE: pleuritic chest pain or breathlessness consistent with PE

TREATMENT CONSIDERATIONS
- Bleeding: contraindication to oral anticoagulation

Examination

CONFIRM THE DIAGNOSIS OF DVT
- Calf swelling (10 cm below the tibial tuberosity) >3 cm difference
- Superficial venous engorgement and pitting oedema

ELLICIT A CAUSE
- Examine abdomen and pelvis (exclude mass compressing veins)

SIGNS OF COMPLICATIONS
- Thrombophlebitis: local tenderness and erythema
- Pulmonary embolus: pleural rub and right heart failure

TREATMENT CONSIDERATIONS
- Peripheral pulses for compression stockings

Discussion

INVESTIGATIONS
- D-dimer (sensitive but not specific test – can rule out diagnosis if negative in low/ intermediate risk cases)
- Doppler/compression ultrasound if D-dimer elevated
- Consider further investigations if an underlying cause is suspected/possible:
  - Thrombophilia screen if recurrent or positive family history
  - CT abdomen/pelvis if aged >50 years
  - Mammography in females
  - PR and PSA in men

TREATMENT
- Anticoagulation: 3 months if provoked, 6 months if unprovoked, lifelong if recurrent/ high risk
- Compression stockings reduce post-phlebitic syndrome

Altered conscious state

This male with diabetes mellitus has been found in a drowsy and confused state.

Diagnosis: diabetic ketoacidosis
Differential diagnosis: meningitis and alcohol/drug intoxication

History

SYMPTOMS (FROM A WITNESS/RELATIVE)

- Polyuria and polydipsia
- Preceding acute illness/fever
- Recent high glucometer readings/increased insulin requirement
- Associated symptoms: nausea, sweating and breathlessness

RISK FACTORS FOR DIABETIC KETOACIDOSIS

- Poor compliance with insulin: young, change in social circumstances

DIFFERENTIAL DIAGNOSIS

- Smelling of alcohol (take care not ketotic), history of drug abuse
- Alcohol and drug history

Examination

CONFIRMATION OF DIAGNOSIS

- Determine Glasgow Coma Score
- Breath: 'pear-drops' (ketones)
- Hyperventilation or Kussmaul's breathing: metabolic acidosis
- Medic alert bracelet/finger prick marks: diabetes

PRECIPITATING FACTORS

- **4 I's** – Insulin forgotten, Infection, Infarction and Injury

COMPLICATIONS

- Retina: diabetic changes, papilloedema
- Pulse and BP: haemodynamic compromise
- Auscultate chest: aspiration pneumonia
  - Gastroparesis due to diabetic autonomic neuropathy

Discussion

INVESTIGATIONS

- Finger-prick glucometer
- Urine dipstick and finger-prick for ketones
- ABG:
  - Metabolic acidosis with respiratory compensation ($\downarrow PaCO_2$)
  - Monitor response to treatment with venous HCO_3^-
- FBC, U&E, LFT and glucose
- ECG (silent MI)
- Blood and urine cultures (sepsis)
- CXR (pneumonia or aspiration)

TREATMENT

- ABC:
  - May require intubation and ITU support
- Fluid resuscitation: crystalloid:
  - Consider K^+ supplementation
- IV insulin sliding scale
- Consider:
  - NG tube to prevent aspiration
  - S/C heparin for VTE prophylaxis
  - Antibiotics for infection

Anaemia
This housebound elderly woman has become more anaemic.

Diagnosis: iron deficiency anaemia (dietary)
Differential diagnosis: chronic GI bleeding; coeliac; inherited haemo-globinopathy, e.g. β-thalassaemia trait

History
SYMPTOMS OF ANAEMIA
- Tiredness, lethargy and breathlessness
- Angina
  Gastrointestinal
  - Stools: altered bowel habit, foul smelling (steatorrhoea), tarry (malaena)
  - Weight loss
  - Indigestion history, GORD, dysphagia and use of NSAIDs
  - Abdominal pain/bloating and wheat intolerance (coeliac)
  Previous history
  - Surgery: small bowel resection or peptic ulcer
  - Inflammatory bowel disease and polyps
  - Menstruation: heavy periods or PV bleeding
  Family history
  - GI malignancy
  - Anaemia: Mediterranean – thalassaemia, Afro-Caribbean – sickle cell
  Travel history
  - Hookworm or tropical sprue
  Planning treatment
- Previous blood transfusions/transfusion reactions

Examination
CONFIRM ANAEMIA
- General pallor
- Pale conjunctivae

DETERMINE CAUSE OF ANAEMIA
- Nails: koilonychia (iron deficiency)
- Mouth: glossitis, angular stomatitis (iron and vitamin B deficiency)
- Sentinel cervical lymph node
- Abdominal mass and hepatomegaly (GI malignancy), epigastric tenderness
- Abdominal scars: small bowel, colon resection
- Offer to perform rectal and vaginal examinations

DETERMINE EFFECT OF ANAEMIA
- Pulse and BP: haemodynamic stability

Discussion
Dietary deficiency causing anaemia is a diagnosis of exclusion

INVESTIGATIONS
- Full blood count: microcytic anaemia and target cells:
  - Iron↓, ferritin↓, total iron binding capacity↑ (folate and vitamin B_{12})
  - Haemoglobin electrophoresis:
    - Thalassaemia and HbE
- Faecal occult blood

- Endoscopy: gastroscopy and colonoscopy
- CT abdomen/barium studies

TREATMENT
- Treat the cause
- Dietary advice and iron supplementation
- Blood transfusion indicated only in extremis (transfusion trigger Hb <70 g/L)

Osler–Weber–Rendu syndrome (hereditary haemorrhagic telangiectasia)

Clinical signs
- Multiple telangiectasia on the face, lips and buccal mucosa

Extra points
- Anaemia: gastrointestinal bleeding
- Cyanosis and chest bruit: pulmonary vascular abnormality/shunt

Discussion
- Autosomal dominant
- Increased risk gastrointestinal haemorrhage, epistaxis and haemoptysis
- Vascular malformations:
  - Pulmonary shunts
  - Intracranial aneurysms: subarachnoid haemorrhage

Haemoptysis
This 74 year-old smoker has had a blood-stained cough.

Diagnosis: bronchial carcinoma
Differential diagnosis: pulmonary embolus, pneumonia, pulmonary oedema

History
SYMPTOMS SUGGESTIVE OF MALIGNANCY
- Cough: chronicity, mucous colour and blood
- Breathlessness
- Chest pain: pleuritic
- General: weight loss (cachexia), bone pain (metastasis) and tiredness (anaemia)
- Rare manifestations of CA bronchus, e.g. paraneoplastic neuropathy
- Abdominal pain: liver metastases or hypercalcaemia
- Headache: brain metastasis

RISK FACTORS
- Smoking history:
  - Calculate number of pack years (20 years' smoking 40 cigarettes/day = 40 pack years)
- Occupation: industrial chemicals, coal dust.

DIFFERENTIAL DIAGNOSIS
- Risk factors for DVT/PE
- Past medical history of ischaemic heart disease and CCF
- Constitutional symptoms: fever and productive cough

Examination
PERIPHERAL STIGMATA OF BRONCHIAL CARCINOMA
- Cachexia
- Nail clubbing and tar-stained fingers (smoking)
- Tattoos from previous radiotherapy

RESPIRATORY EXAMINATION
- Cervical lymphadenopathy
- Tracheal deviation: lobar collapse
- Dull percussion note: consolidation and effusion
- Reduced air entry/bronchial breathing

METASTASES
- Craggy hepatomegaly
- Spinal tenderness on percussion with heel of hand
- Focal neurology: cerebral

Discussion
INVESTIGATION
- CXR: mass, pleural effusion and bone erosion
- CT chest/staging CT
- Bronchoscopy/CT-guided biopsy or lymph biopsy/excision: tissue diagnosis

TREATMENT
- Surgical: lobectomy
- Medical:
  - Chemotherapy: cisplatin/gemcitabine
  - Radiotherapy
  - Palliative care

Worsening mobility

Please can you assess this 87-year-old woman who has worsening mobility.

Diagnosis: UTI
Differential diagnosis: drug side effects, pneumonia and stroke

History

PRE-MORBID SOCIAL HISTORY
* Independence → dependence (identify carer role/frequency)
* Mobility issues: Parkinsonism, stroke etc.:
  o Unaided → stick → frame
  o Falls recently
* Housing (important for discharge planning)

PRECIPITANT
* Infection:
  o Urinary symptoms: dysuria, frequency and incontinence
  o Pneumonia: cough and breathlessness
* Drug changes recently: benzodiazepines (sleepiness), diuretics and BP medication (postural hypotension), antipsychotic (extrapyramidal side effects), steroids (proximal myopathy), anti-parkinsonian drug changes
* Systemic enquiry: sites of pain

LEGAL ASPECTS
* Advanced directives or living wills
* Power of attorney
* DNAR and other treatments

Examination
* A lot of information can be obtained by asking the patient to stand and walk unaided (ensure patient safety):
  o Proximal lower limb motor strength: rising from a chair
  o Gait: wide based/ataxic (cerebellar), hemiplegic (stroke) and shuffling (Parkinson's syndrome)
  o Romberg's sign:
    o Positive if patient stumbles forward on closing his or her eyes (protect the patient from falling when assessing this)
    o Balance requires sensory input from at least two sources: vision, vestibular and proprioception
* If bed bound assess lower limbs:
  o Inspection: wasting
  o Tone: ankle clonus
  o Power: 'lift foot off the bed'
  o Coordination: 'run your heel up and down the shin of your other leg'
  o Reflexes: knee jerk and plantar jerks
* Postural dizziness:
  o Assess lying and standing BP:
    o >20 mm Hg drop in systolic BP (at 2 minutes) is significant

Discussion
INVESTIGATIONS
* Sepsis screen: urine, blood cultures and CXR
* If fall and altered conscious state/confusion consider CT head:
  o Subdural haematoma: especially in atrophic brain

MANAGEMENT
- Treat reversible causes: antibiotics, avoid poly-pharmacy
- MDT case conference: nurse, social worker, occupational therapy and physiotherapy:
  - Stick/frame
  - Home improvements or residential care
  - Resuscitation decision

Persistent fever

Please assess this young man with fever and malaise for the last 3 months.

Diagnosis: infection (endocarditis)
Differential diagnosis: drug-induced, malignancy (lymphoma) and inflammatory disease

History
INFECTION
- Temporal pattern:
  ○ Fever at night: malaria
- Contacts:
  ○ TB
- SH:
  ○ Foreign travel:
    ○ Malarial regions
  ○ Sexual:
    ○ HIV risk
  ○ Drug abuse:
    ○ Endocarditis and HIV risk
  ○ Psychiatric history/stress (factitious):
    ○ Medical professional

DRUG
- After change in medication (drug-induced)
- Malignant hyperpyrexia syndrome:
  ○ Antipsychotic medication
  ○ Associated with muscle pain
- Allergies to antibiotic and antibiotic history

MALIGNANCY
- Weight loss
- Lumps: painless lymphadenopathy (lymphoma and HIV)
- Smoker, breathlessness and chest pain (lung)
- Altered bowel habit (colon)

INFLAMMATORY
- Joint or skin problems

Examination
PERIPHERAL
- Look for needle tracks
- Splinter haemorrhages (fingers)
- Roth spots (fundoscopy)
- Lymphadenopathy

CARDIOVASCULAR
- Murmur: endocarditis

ABDOMINAL EXAMINATION
- Craggy liver or mass (malignancy)
- Splenomegaly (infection, inflammatory and malignancy)
- Dip the urine: haematuria (endocarditis)

JOINTS, SKIN AND EYES
- Inflammatory conditions

Discussion

INVESTIGATION

- Septic screen:
  - Blood including repeated thick and thin film (parasitaemia)
  - Urine, bone marrow aspirate and CSF
  - HIV testing
- CRP, ESR, autoantibodies, immunoglobulins and complement levels
- CK (malignant hyperthermia)
- TOE: vegetations, aortic root abscess and myxoma

MANAGEMENT

- Avoid early antibiotics until identification of the cause
- Consider stopping all drugs and reinstituting them one-by-one
- Admit the patient and monitor them closely:
  - Fever that resolves during close observation may be factitious!

Dyspnoea

Please assess this young woman with sudden onset breathlessness.

Diagnosis: asthma
Differential diagnosis: PE and pneumothorax

History

ASTHMA

- Sudden-onset wheeze, short of breath and cough (non-productive)
- Triggers
  - Allergy:
    - Pets, food, dust and pollen
    - Atopic: allergic rhinitis and eczema
    - Anaphylaxis
    - Allergy-testing clinic
  - Upper respiratory tract infection:
    - Sore throat, fever, etc.
- Severity:
  - ITU admissions (brittle asthma):
    - Intubation risk
- Drug history:
  - Compliance with preventor medication
  - Inhaler technique
  - EpiPen

DIFFERENTIAL DIAGNOSIS

- Pneumothorax:
  - Spontaneous in asthmatics or tall, thin individuals
  - Permanent pacemaker or central line
- Symptoms and risk factors for DVT causing PE

Examination

SEVERITY (DOES THIS PATIENT NEED ITU?)

- Conscious level
- Respiratory rate:
  - Count 1–10: how far do they get on one breath?
- Pulse and blood pressure

RESPIRATORY

- Expansion and percussion note increased bilaterally due to lung hyper-expansion:
  - Unilateral (pneumothorax)
- Polyphonic wheeze:
  - Silent chest is a sign of severity
- Stridor, angioedema and tongue swelling (anaphylaxis)

SKIN

- Urticaria (anaphylaxis)

DIFFERENTIAL DIAGNOSIS

- Unilateral reduced air entry, reduced breath sounds and increased resonance on percussion (pneumothorax):
  - Tracheal and/or apex beat deviation away (tension pneumothorax)
- Calf swelling (DVT → PE)

Discussion

INVESTIGATIONS

- Arterial blood gas:
  - Hypoxaemia
  - Normal or rising $PaCO_2$ suggests a tiring patient requiring respiratory support (should have a respiratory alkalosis)
- CXR in exhalation (pneumothorax)

TREATMENT

- Asthma:
  - Bronchodilators and steroids (not routine antibiotics as often viral)
  - Asthma specialist nurse:
    - Inhaler technique
  - Allergy clinic
- Pneumothorax:
  - Needle aspiration or chest drain
  - May need talc or surgical pleurodesis if it is recurrent

Syncope
Please evaluate this 75-year-old woman who blacked-out at the dinner table without warning.

History
- Description of the syncopal episode:
  - Provocation: micturation, cough or stressful situation (vasovagal)
  - Prodrome: light headed, dizziness, tunnel vision (vasovagal/orthostatic), no warning (cardiac)
  - Posture: sitting/lying (cardiac) or standing (orthostatic), sudden head turning (vertebrobasilar)
  - Associated symptoms: palpitations and chest pain (cardiac), headache, tongue biting and incontinence (neuro)
  - Duration (transient, <5 minutes) and frequency
  - Recovery: immediate (cardiac) or prolonged confused state and amnesia (>5 minutes) (neuro), red/flushed face (cardiac)
  - Injury (neuro or cardiac)
  - Eyewitness account is very useful
- Past medical history of syncope/presyncope, cardiac disease or neurological conditions
- Medications that may cause hypotension

Examination
- Brief cardiovascular exam
  - Pulse and blood pressure (lying and standing), postural drop: >20/10 mm Hg difference
  - Auscultation: obstructive valvular pathology e.g. AS or MS or signs of a PE (loud P_2 and left parasternal heave)
  - Pacemaker or ICD scars
- Brief neurological exam
  - Fundoscopy
  - Pronator drift
  - Reflexes
  - Parkinson's plus tremor, rigidity, bradykinesia and orthostatic hypotension, e.g. multiple system atrophy

Discussion
- Differential diagnosis:
  - Cardiac: brady- or tachycardia, obstructive cardiac lesion: AS, MS, HOCM or PE
  - Neurological: epilepsy, vertebrobasilar insufficiency
  - Orthostatic (postural) hypotension: particularly in combination with vasodilator drugs
  - Vasovagal (neurocardiogenic): stress, cough, micturation, defecation
- Investigation
  - 12-lead ECG, Holter monitor, implantable loop recorder, electrophysiology study, ETT and Echo if cardiac cause suspected
  - Tilt table test if orthostatic hypotension suspected
  - EEG and/or CT MRI brain if a neurological cause is suspected
- Management
  - Cardiac: pacemaker, ICD, revascularisation and valvular surgery
  - Vasovagal: education on avoidance, isotonic muscle contraction

- o Orthostatic hypotension: salt and water replacement, support stockings, medication review, occasionally fludrocortisone, midodrine, SSRIs and pacemaker are helpful
- o Neurological: antiepileptic medication
- DVLA (Group 1 license: car/motorbike)
  - o Check the 3 P's: **p**rovocation/**p**rodrome/**p**ostural – if all present then likely benign and can continue driving.
  - o Solitary with no clear cause – 6 month ban; clear cause that has been treated – resume driving after 4 weeks
  - o Recurrent syncope due to seizures – must be fit free for 1 year to drive.

Atrial fibrillation

This 81-year-old gentleman has had intermittent palpitations and breathlessness and noticed transient left facial and upper-arm paraesthesia.

History
- Symptoms of atrial fibrillation
  - Onset and offset, frequency and duration
  - Breathlessness, chest pain, palpitations, presyncope
  - Precipitants: alcohol, caffeine, exercise
- Associated conditions
  - Cardiac problems: valvular heart disease
  - Hypertension
  - Hyperthyroidism
  - Stroke or TIA (likely in this case)
  - Lung disease including PE
- Treatment consideration
  - Anticoagulation and risk factors for bleeding
  - Anti-arrhythmic vs cardioversion vs pulmonary vein isolation

Examination
- Cardiovascular examination
  - Pulse and BP
  - Auscultation: murmurs – MS or MR
  - Signs of CCF
- Assessment of thyroid status
  - Tremor
  - Goitre
  - Eye disease: lid lag, exophthalmos (Grave's disease)
- Brief neurological examination
  - Pronator drift
  - Visual fields
  - CN VII weakness
  - CN V and upper limb sensation
  - Gait

Discussion
- Investigations:
  - Confirmation: 12-lead ECG or 24-hour Holter monitor
  - Echo: structural disease, LVH, LA size (>4.0 cm – recurrence high)
  - TSH
- Types
  - Paroxysmal: <7 days, self terminating
  - Persistent: >7 days, requires chemical or electrical cardioversion
  - Permanent: >1 year or when no further attempts to restore sinus
- Management:
  - Rhythm control: chemical or electrical cardioversion
  - Rate control: β-blockers, digoxin, pacemaker and AVN ablation
- Pulmonary vein isolation: reserved for refractory, symptomatic patients
  - More successful in paroxysmal AF (>90% cure rate)
  - Young: to limit progression to permanent AF
- Anticoagulation: warfarin or novel oral anticoagulants (NOACs)
- Risk prediction:
  Embolic risk equivalent for paroxysmal, persistent and permanent AF

Systemic emboli risk:

C   Congestive cardiac failure = 1
H   Hypertension = 1
A_2 Age ≥75 = 2
D   Diabetes = 1
S_2 Stroke/TIA/embolus = 2
V   Vascular disease = 1
A   Age 65–74 = 1
Sc   Sex category (female) = 1

0 = Low stroke risk = no anticoagulation
1 = Medium stroke risk (1.3% per annum) = patient preference
≥2 = High risk (>2.2% per annum) = oral anticoagulation recommended

Bleeding risk:

H   Hypertension = 1
A   Abnormal kidney or liver function = 1 for each
S   Stroke = 1
B   Bleeding = 1
L   Labile INR = 1
E   Elderly = 1
D   Drugs (NSAIDs) and alcohol = 1 for each

≥3 = high risk (avoid oral anticoagulation)

Patients high risk for both embolic and bleeding complications should be considered for left atrial appendage occlusion to isolate the commonest source of thrombus in AF.

- Prevalence: 8% of >80-year-olds have AF

Inflammatory bowel disease

This 36-year-old male has had bloody diarrhoea intermittently for the past 6 weeks. He has lost about 3 kg in weight.

History
- Gastrointestinal symptoms
  - Duration
  - Precipitants (travel, antibiotics, infectious contacts, foods, sexual history)
  - Stool frequency and consistency (Bristol stool scale)
  - Blood: fresh PR/mixed with stools
  - Mucus/slime
  - Urgency, incontinence, tenesmus
  - Abdominal pain, bloating: and association with eating, defecation
- Systemic symptoms
  - Fever
  - Anorexia
  - Weight loss
  - Rash, arthralgia, aphthous ulcers
- Family history

Examination
- General
  - Pallor/anaemia
  - Nutritional status
  - Pulse and BP
  - Oral ulceration
- Abdomen
  - Surgical scars, including current/past stoma sites
  - Tenderness
  - Palpable masses (e.g. right iliac fossa mass in Crohn's disease or colonic tumour in UC)
  - Ask to examine for perianal disease
- Evidence of treatment
  - Steroid side effects
  - Ciclosporin (gum hypertrophy and hypertension)
  - Hickman lines/scars

Discussion
- Investigations
  - Stool microscopy and culture: exclude infective cause of diarrhoea
  - FBC and inflammatory markers: monitor disease activity
  - AXR: exclude toxic dilatation in UC and small bowel obstruction due to strictures in Crohn's
  - Sigmoidoscopy/colonoscopy and biopsy: histological confirmation
  - Bowel contrast studies: strictures and fistulae in Crohn's disease
  - Further imaging: white cell scan and CT scan
- Cause
  - Genetic, environmental and other factors combine to produce an exaggerated, sustained and mucosal inflammatory response
- Differential diagnosis
  - Crohn's: *Yersinia*, tuberculosis, lymphoma (and UC)
  - UC: infection (e.g. campylobacter), ischaemia, drugs and radiation (and Crohn's)

- Treatment
  - Medical

	Crohn's	**UC**
Mild–moderate disease	Oral steroid (5-ASA)	Oral or topical (rectal steroid) 5-ASA (e.g. mesalazine)
Severe disease	IV steroid IV infliximab	IV steroid IV ciclosporin
Maintenance therapy	Oral steroid Azathioprine Methotrexate TNFα inhibitors: Infliximab, adalimumab	Oral steroid 5-ASA Azathioprine

  - Antibiotics (metronidazole): in Crohn's with perianal infection, fistulae or small bowel bacterial overgrowth
  - Nutritional support: high fibre, elemental and low residue diets
  - Psychological support
  - Surgery
    - Crohn's: obstruction from strictures, complications from fistulae and perianal disease and failure to respond to medical therapy
    - UC: chronic symptomatic relief, emergency surgery for severe refractory colitis and colonic dysplasia or carcinoma
- Complications

Crohn's disease	Ulcerative colitis
Malabsorption	Anaemia
Anaemia	Toxic dilatation
Abscess	Perforation
Fistula	Colonic
Intestinal obstruction	carcinoma

- Colonic carcinoma and UC
  - Higher risk in patients with pancolitis (5–10% at 15–20 years), and in those with PSC
  - Surveillance: 3-yearly colonoscopy for patients with pancolitis >10 years, increasing in frequency with every decade from diagnosis (2-yearly 20–30 years, annually >30 years)
  - Colectomy if dysplasia is detected
- Extra-intestinal manifestations

Mouth:	Apthous ulcers*
Skin:	Erythema nodosum*
	Pyoderma gangrenosum*
	Finger clubbing*
Joint:	Large joint arthritis*
	Seronegative arthritides
Eye:	Uveitis*, episcleritis* and iritis*
Liver:	Primary sclerosing cholangitis (UC)
Systemic amyloidosis	

(*related to disease activity)

Hypertension

This 37-year-old woman presented with intermittent headaches for the past 3 months. Her blood pressure is elevated – I would be grateful for your opinion.

History
- Duration of symptoms, nature of headache
- Past history of hypertension: previous blood pressure readings (e.g. employment medical, with prescription of oral contraceptive pill, during pregnancy)
- Other medical history (e.g. renal disease), cardiovascular risk factors (smoking, diabetes, known ischaemic heart disease)
- Drug history (prescribed and illicit), alcohol consumption
- Visual disturbance (in accelerated phase hypertension)
- Paroxysomal symptoms (phaeochromocytoma)
- Check if pregnant!

Examination
- Body habitus: obese, Cushingoid, acromegalic
- Radial pulse (SR/AF), radio-radial and radio-femoral delay (coarctation)
- Check the blood pressure yourself, with a manual sphygmomanometer, in both arms
- Evidence of cardiac failure
- Underlying renal cause: renal bruit(s), polycystic kidney disease, current renal replacement therapy (dialysis/transplant), ask to dip the urine
- Fundoscopy: hypertensive retinopathy

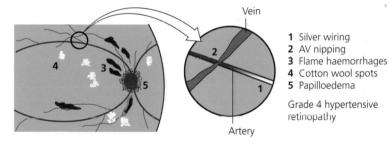

Vein

1 Silver wiring
2 AV nipping
3 Flame haemorrhages
4 Cotton wool spots
5 Papilloedema

Grade 4 hypertensive retinopathy

Artery

- ○ Grade 1: silver wiring (increased reflectance from thickened arterioles)
- ○ Grade 2: plus arteriovenous nipping (narrowing of veins as arterioles cross them)
- ○ Grade 3: plus cotton wool spots and flame haemorrhages
- ○ Grade 4: plus papilloedema
- There may also be hard exudates (macular star)

Discussion

CAUSES OF HYPERTENSION
- Essential (94%: associated with age, obesity, salt and alcohol)
- Renal (4%: underlying chronic kidney disease secondary to glomerulonephritis, ADPKD, renovascular disease)
- Endocrine (1%: Conn's, Cushing's, acromegaly or phaeochromocytoma)
- Aortic coarctation
- Pre-eclampsia: pregnancy

INVESTIGATION
- Evidence of end-organ damage: fundoscopy, LVH on ECG, renal impairment, cardiac failure on CXR, echocardiography
- Exclude underlying cause:
  - ○ Urine pregnancy test (where appropriate!)
  - ○ Urinalysis (and urine ACR)

- o U&Es
- o Consider secondary screen: renin/aldosterone levels, plasma and/or urinary metanephrines

DIAGNOSIS
- Current (2011) British Hypertension Society guidelines:
  - o Clinic BP >140/90 mm Hg: use 24 h ABPM to confirm diagnosis (average of daytime values)
  - o Definitions;
    - o Stage 1 hypertension: clinic BP ≥140/90 mm Hg or ABPM daytime average ≥135/85 mm Hg
    - o Stage 2 hypertension: clinic BP ≥160/100 mm Hg or ABPM daytime average ≥150/95 mm Hg
    - o Severe hypertension: clinic SBP ≥180 mm Hg or DBP ≥110 mm Hg
  - o Treat if stage 1 hypertension and evidence of end-organ damage, ischaemic heart disease, diabetes, CKD or 10-year cardiovascular risk ≥20%
  - o Treat all with stage 2 hypertension
- Arrange same-day admission if severe hypertension and grade 3 or 4 retinopathy (or other concerns; e.g. new renal impairment)

TREATMENT
- Lifestyle modification (lose weight, increase exercise, stop smoking)
- Initial treatment:
  - o ACE-I or ARB
  - o Aged >55 years or Afro-Caribbean ethnicity: CCB or thiazide-like diuretic
  - o Titrate dose to maximum tolerated
- Then add CCB or thiazide-like diuretic
- Then ACE-I/ARB + CCB + thiazide-like diuretic
- Consider adding spironolactone, β-blocker, α-blocker or seeking specialist opinion
- Consider other cardiovascular risk modification: aspirin, statin

ACCELERATED PHASE ('MALIGNANT') HYPERTENSION
- Medical emergency

Treatment
- Grade III and IV retinopathy and hypertension
  - o Bed rest, oral anti-hypertensives (long-acting CCB) and non-invasive blood pressure monitoring: aiming for gradual reduction in blood pressure
- Plus encephalopathy/stroke/myocardial infarction/left ventricular failure.
  - o Parenteral venodilators and invasive blood pressure monitoring.
  - o Over-rapid fall in blood pressure can lead to 'watershed' cerebral and retinal infarction.

Papilloedema
Blurring of disc margins/elevation of disc/loss of venous pulsation/venous engorgement

CAUSES
- Raised intracranial pressure: space-occupying lesion, benign intracranial hypertension and cavernous sinus thrombosis
- Accelerated phase hypertension
- Central retinal vein occlusion

DIFFERENTIAL DIAGNOSIS
Papilloedema: normal visual acuity, obscurations and tunnel vision. Usually bilateral
Papillitis: reduced visual acuity, central scotoma and pain. Usually unilateral. Seen with inflammation of the head of the optic nerve; e.g. in mitral stenosis

Red rashes
This patient has a rash.

Diagnosis: psoriasis
History
DESCRIBE THE RASH
- Location, appearance, pruritis

PSYCHOSOCIAL IMPACT
- Particularly important in young women
- Confidence, relationships, work
- Depression

EXACERBATING FACTORS
- Stress, alcohol, cigarettes, drugs (β-blockers), trauma

TREATMENT
- PUVA: risk of melanoma (fair skin, family history)
- Immunosuppression: intercurrent infections
- Systemic side-effects: steroids
- Pregnancy? Some treatments are teratogenic

Examination
SKIN
- Chronic plaque (classical) type: multiple, well-demarcated, 'salmon-pink', scaly plaques on **extensor** surface
- Check behind ears, scalp and umbilicus
- Koebner phenomenon: plaques at sites of trauma
- Skin staining from treatment

NAILS
- Pitting, onycholysis, hyperkeratosis, discoloration

JOINTS
- **Psoriatic arthropathy** (10%), five forms:
  - DIPJ involvement (similar to OA)
  - Large joint mono/oligoarthritis
  - Seronegative (similar to RA)
  - Sacroilitis (similar to ankylosing spondylitis)
  - Arthritis mutilans

Discussion
DEFINITION
Epidermal hyperproliferation and accumulation of inflammatory cells

TREATMENT
Topical (in- or outpatient)

- **Emollients**
- **Calcipotriol**
- **Coal tar**
  - Stains brown
- **Dithranol**
  - Stains purple and burns normal skin
- **Hydrocortisone**

PHOTOTHERAPY
- UVB
- Psoralen + UVA (PUVA)

SYSTEMIC
- **Cytotoxics** (methotrexate and ciclosporin)
- **Anti-TNFα** (adalimumab: Humira)
- **Retinoids** (Acitretin): teratogenic

COMPLICATIONS
- **Erythroderma**: life-threatening

CAUSES OF NAIL PITTING
- **Psoriasis**
- Lichen planus
- Alopecia areata
- Fungal infections

KOEBNER PHENOMENON SEEN WITH
- **Psoriasis**
- Lichen planus
- Viral warts
- Vitiligo
- Sarcoid

Diagnosis: eczema
History
DESCRIBE THE RASH
- Location, appearance, pruritis

PSYCHOSOCIAL IMPACT
- Particularly important in young women
- Confidence, relationships, work
- Depression

ATOPIC (ENDOGENOUS)
- Asthma, hay fever and allergy

ENVIRONMENTAL (EXOGENOUS)
- Primary irritant dermatitis: may just affect hands
- What is their job?

Examination
RASH
- Erythematous and lichenified patches of skin
- Predominantly **flexor** aspects of joints
- Fissures (painful), especially hands and feet
- Excoriations
- Secondary bacterial infection

ASSOCIATED ATOPY
- Respiratory: polyphonic wheeze (asthma)

SYSTEMIC TREATMENT EFFECTS
- Steroids: e.g. blood pressure

Discussion
INVESTIGATIONS
- Patch testing for allergies

TREATMENT
- Avoid precipitants
- Topical:
  ○ Emollients
  ○ Steroids
  ○ Tacrolimus (protopic): small increased risk of Bowen's disease
- Anti-histamines for pruritis
- Antibiotics for secondary infection
- UV light therapy
- Systemic therapy (prednisolone) in severe cases

Leg ulcers

I'm worried about this man's leg ulcers.

Diagnosis: venous leg ulcer
Differential: arterial or diabetic (neuropathic) leg ulcer

History

DESCRIBE SYMPTOMS
- Pain: arterial (venous and neuropathic are painless)
- Location

ASSOCIATED DISEASES
- Venous: DVT, chronic venous insufficiency, varicose veins, CCF
- Arterial: PVD
- Neuropathic: sensory neuropathy, diabetes

COMPLICATIONS
- Systemic signs of infection

Examination

VENOUS
- Gaiter area of lower leg
- **Stigmata of venous hypertension**: varicose veins or scars from vein stripping, oedema, lipodermatosclerosis, varicose eczema, atrophie blanche
- **Pelvic/abdominal mass**

ARTERIAL
- Distal extremities and pressure points
- Trophic changes: hairless and paper-thin shiny skin
- Cold with poor capillary refill
- **Absent distal pulses**

NEUROPATHIC
- Pressure areas, e.g. under the metatarsal heads
- **Peripheral neuropathy**
- Charcot's joints

COMPLICATIONS
- **Infection:** temperature, pus and cellulites
- **Malignant change:** Marjolin's ulcer (squamous cell carcinoma)

Discussion

OTHER CAUSES OF A LEG ULCER
- Vasculitic, e.g. rheumatoid arthritis
- Neoplastic, e.g. squamous cell carcinoma
- Infectious, e.g. syphilis
- Haematological, e.g. sickle cell anaemia
- Tropical, e.g. cutaneous leishmaniasis

INVESTIGATIONS
- Doppler ultrasound
- Ankle–brachial pressure index (0.8–1.2 is normal, <0.8 implies arterial insufficiency)
- Arteriography

TREATMENT
Specialist nurse: wound care
Venous
- Four-layer compression bandaging (if no PVD)
- Varicose vein surgery

Arterial
- Angioplasty or vascular reconstruction/amputation

CAUSES OF NEUROPATHIC ULCERS
- Diabetes mellitus
- Tabes dorsalis
- Syringomyelia

Diabetes and the skin

This 32-year-old female has had type I diabetes mellitus for many years and now has a rash on her legs.

Diagnosis: necrobiosis lipoidica diabeticorum
Differential: diabetic dermopathy, granuloma annulare, leg ulcers, eruptive xanthomata, vitiligo, candidiasis

History

DIABETIC HISTORY/CARE
- Duration
- Insulin administration and glucose control: rotation of injection sites
- Foot care: podiatry

MICROVASCULAR COMPLICATIONS OF DIABETES
- Neuropathy
- Retinopathy

PSYCHOSOCIAL
- Impact on ability to work, form relationships, body image

Examination

SHINS
- Necrobiosis lipoidica diabeticorum:
  - Well-demarcated plaques with waxy-yellow centre and red–brown edges
  - Early: may resemble a bruise
  - Prominent skin blood vessels
  - Female preponderance (90%)
- Diabetic dermopathy:
  - Red/brown, atrophic lesions

FEET AND LEGS
- Ulcers: arterial or neuropathic (see Leg ulcers section, p. 146)
- Eruptive xanthomata:
  - Yellow papules on buttocks and knees (also elbows)
  - Caused by hyperlipidaemia
- Granuloma annulare: flesh-coloured papules in annular configurations on the dorsum feet (and more commonly fingers)

INJECTION SITES (THIGH)
- Lipoatrophy
- Fat hypertrophy

CUTANEOUS INFECTIONS
- Cellulitis
- Candidiasis (intertrigo): in skin creases

OTHER DISEASES
- Vitiligo (and other autoimmune diseases)
- PVD: pulses

Discussion

TREATMENT FOR NECROBIOSIS LIPOIDICA DIABETICORUM
- Topical steroid and support bandaging
- Tight glycaemic control does not help

XANTHOMATA

- **Hypercholesterolaemia:** tendon xanthomata, xanthelasma and corneal arcus
- **Hypertriglyceridaemia:** eruptive xanthomata and lipaemia retinalis
- **Other causes of secondary hyperlipidaemia:**
  - Hypothyroidism
  - Nephrotic syndrome
  - Alcohol
  - Cholestasis

Erythema nodosum
History
SKIN
- Tender, red, smooth, shiny nodules on the shins

CAUSES
- Sarcoidosis
- Streptococcal throat infection
- Streptomycin, sulphonamides
- Oral contraceptive pill
- Pregnancy
- TB
- Inflammatory bowel disease
- Lymphoma
- Idiopathic

Examination
SKIN
- Tender, red, smooth, shiny nodules commonly found on the shins (although anywhere with subcutaneous fat)
- Older lesions leave a bruise

JOINTS
- Tenderness and swelling

CAUSE
- Red, sore throat (streptococcal infection)
- Parotid swelling (sarcoidosis)

Discussion
- Pathology: inflammation of subcutaneous fat (panniculitis)

Other skin manifestations of sarcoidosis:

- **Nodules and papules:** red/brown seen particularly around the face, nose, ears and neck. Demonstrates Koebner's phenomenon
- **Lupus pernio:** diffuse bluish/brown plaque with central small papules commonly affecting the nose

Henoch–Schönlein purpura
History
TRIAD
- Purpuric rash: usually on buttocks and legs
- Arthritis
- Abdominal pain

PRECIPITANTS
- Infections: streptococci, HSV, parvovirus B19, etc.
- Drugs: antibiotics

COMPLICATIONS
- Renal involvement (IgA nephropathy): visible or non-visible haematuria, proteinuria
- Hypertension

Examination
RASH
- Purpuric rash: usually on buttocks and legs

JOINTS
- Arthritis

OTHER
- Blood pressure
- Urine dipstick

Discussion
- Small-vessel vasculitis: IgA and C3 deposition
- Normal or raised platelet count (distinguishes from other forms of purpura)
- Children more than adults, males > females
- Treatment: most spontaneously recover without treatment although steroids may help recovery and treat painful arthralgia
- Prognosis: 90% full recovery although can recur

Skin malignancy
This patient has noticed a lump on their face.

Diagnosis: basal cell carcinoma
Differential: malignant melanoma, squamous cell carcinoma, actinic keratosis

History
SYMPTOMS
- Location and rapidity of growth
- Recent changes or bleeding

RISK FACTORS
- Sun exposure
- Occupation: exposure to dust/chemicals, outdoor work
- Family or past medical history of skin cancer

ASSOCIATIONS
- Solid organ transplant: immunosuppression

COMPLICATIONS
- Local invasion or metastasis: bone pain, neurological or abdominal problems

Basal cell carcinoma
- Usually on face/trunk: sun-exposed areas
- Pearly nodule with rolled edge
- Superficial telangiectasia
- Ulceration in advanced lesions
- Other lesions

NATURAL HISTORY
- Slowly grow over a few months
- Local invasion only, rarely metastasize

TREATMENT
- Curettage/cryotherapy if superficial
- Surgical excision ± radiotherapy

Squamous cell carcinoma
- Sun-exposed areas (+ lips + mouth)
- Actinic keratoses: pre-malignant (red and scaly patches)
- Varied appearance
  - Keratotic nodule
  - Polypoid mass
  - Cutaneous ulcer
- Other lesions/previous scars
- Metastases (draining lymph nodes/hepatomegaly/bone tenderness)

DISCUSSION
- Squamous cell carcinoma *in situ* (Bowen's disease)

DIAGNOSIS
- Biopsy suspicious lesions

TREATMENT
- Surgery ± radiotherapy
- 5% metastasize

Malignant melanoma
- Patient's appearance: mention risks
  - Fair skin with freckles
  - Light hair
  - Blue eyes
- Appearance of lesion
  Asymmetrical
  Border irregularity
  Colour (black: often irregular pigmentation, may be colourless)
  Diameter >6 mm
  Enlarging
- Other lesions/previous scars
- Metastases (draining lymph nodes/hepatomegaly/bone tenderness)

DIAGNOSIS/TREATMENT
- Excision
- Staged on Breslow thickness (maximal depth of tumour invasion into dermis):
  - <1.5 mm = 90% 5-year survival
  - >3.5 mm = 40% 5-year survival
  Beware the man with a glass eye and ascites: ocular melanoma!

Skin and hyperextensible joints
I'd like to refer this patient with a skin problem.

Pseudoxanthoma elasticum
HISTORY
Explore skin problems
• Hereditary: chronic

Other problems
• Hyperextensible joints
• Reduced visual acuity
• Hypertension
• MI or CVA
• Gastric bleed

Family history

EXAMINATION
Skin
• 'Plucked chicken skin' appearance: loose skin folds especially at the neck and axillae, with yellow pseudoxanthomatous plaques

Eyes
• Blue sclerae
• Retinal angioid streaks (cracks in Bruch's membrane) and macular degeneration

Cardiovascular
• Blood pressure: 50% are hypertensive
• Mitral valve prolapse: EC and PSM

DISCUSSION
• Inheritance: 80% autosomal recessive (*ABCC6* gene, chromosome 16)
• Degenerative elastic fibres in skin, blood vessels and eye
• Premature coronary artery disease

Differential diagnosis: Ehlers–Danlos
HISTORY
• As above
• No premature coronary disease
• Family history more apparent (autosomal dominant)

EXAMINATION
Skin and joints
• Fragile skin: multiple ecchymoses, scarring – 'fish-mouth' scars especially on the knees
• Hyperextensible skin: able to tent up skin when pulled (avoid doing this)
• Joint hypermobility and dislocation (scar from joint repair/replacement)

Cardiac
• Mitral valve prolapse

Abdominal

- Scars:
  - Aneurysmal rupture and dissection
  - Bowel perforation and bleeding

DISCUSSION

- Inheritance: autosomal dominant
- Defect in collagen causing increased skin elasticity
- No premature coronary artery disease

Rheumatoid arthritis
This young woman has had painful, stiff fingers.

History
SYMPTOMS
• Joints involved, pain, function

DISABILITY AND HANDICAP
• Occupation and ADLs

DRUGS
• Will help assess disease activity

SYSTEMIC EFFECTS OF DISEASE AND TREATMENT
• See below

Examination
OBSERVE HANDS (SLEEVES ROLLED BEYOND ELBOW)
• Symmetrical and deforming polyarthropathy
• Volar subluxation and ulnar deviation at the MCPJs
• Subluxation at the wrist
• Swan-neck deformity (hyperextension of the PIPJ and flexion of the DIPJ)
• Boutonnière's deformity (flexion of the PIPJ and hyperextension of the DIPJ)
• 'Z' thumbs
• Muscle wasting (disuse atrophy)
• Surgical scars:
   ○ Carpal tunnel release (wrist)
   ○ Joint replacement (especially thumb)
   ○ Tendon transfer (dorsum of hand)
• Rheumatoid nodules (elbows)

ASSESS DISEASE ACTIVITY
• Red, swollen, hot, painful hands imply active disease

ASSESS FUNCTION
• **Power grip:** 'squeeze my fingers'
• **Precision grip:** 'pick up a coin' or 'do up your buttons'
• **Key grip:** 'pretend to use this key'
• Remember the wheelchair, walking aids and splints

TREATMENT EFFECTS
• Steroids: Cushingoid
• C-spine stabilization scars

SYSTEMIC MANIFESTATIONS OF RA
• **Pulmonary:**
   ○ Pleural effusions
   ○ Fibrosing alveolitis
   ○ Obliterative bronchiolitis
   ○ Caplan's nodules
• **Eyes:**
   ○ Dry (secondary Sjögren's)
   ○ Scleritis

- **Neurological:**
  - Carpal tunnel syndrome (commonest)
  - Atlanto-axial subluxation: quadriplegia
  - Peripheral neuropathy
- **Haematological:**
  - Felty's syndrome: RA + splenomegaly + neutropaenia
  - Anaemia (all types!)
- **Cardiac:**
  - Pericarditis
- **Renal:**
  - Nephrotic syndrome (secondary amyloidosis or membraneous glomerulonephritis, e.g. due to penicillamine)

Main differential diagnosis

- Psoriatic arthropathy:
  - Nail changes
  - Psoriasis: elbows, behind ears and scalp

Discussion

INVESTIGATIONS

- Elevated inflammatory markers
- Radiological changes:
  - Soft tissue swelling
  - Loss of joint space
  - Articular erosions
  - Periarticular osteoporosis
- Positive rheumatoid factor in 80%

DIAGNOSIS: 4/7 OF AMERICAN COLLEGE OF RHEUMATOLOGY CRITERIA

- Morning stiffness
- Arthritis in 3+ joint areas
- Arthritis of hands
- Symmetrical arthritis
- Rheumatoid nodules
- Positive rheumatoid factor
- Erosions on joint radiographs

TREATMENT

Medical

- Symptomatic relief: NSAIDs and COX-2 inhibitors
- Early introduction of disease-modifying anti-rheumatoid drugs (DMARDs) to suppress disease activity:

	Serious side effects	Monitor
Methotrexate	Neutropenia, pulmonary toxicity and hepatitis	CXR, FBC, LFT
Hydroxychloroquine	Retinopathy	Visual acuity
Sulphasalazine	Rash and bone marrow suppression	FBC
Corticosteroids	Osteoporosis	
Azathioprine	Neutropenia	FBC
Gold complexes	Thrombocytopaenia, rash	FBC
Penicillamine	Proteinuria, thrombocytopaenia rash	FBC and urine

Ongoing disease activity may require immunomodulation therapy:
- **Anti-TNF therapy:** Infliximab/Etanercept/Adalimumab:
    - Side effects include rash, opportunistic infection (exclude TB: Heaf test and CXR)
- **B cell depletion therapy:** Rituximab (anti-CD20 mAb)

Supportive
- Explanation and education
- Exercise and physiotherapy
- Occupational therapy and social support

Surgery
- Joint replacement, tendon transfer, etc.

PROGNOSIS
- 5 years – 1/3 unable to work; 10 years – 1/2 significant disability

Systemic lupus erythematosus
Please see this woman with a rash on her face.

History

DESCRIBE THE RASH
- Location, appearance, other areas affected
- Photosensitivity

ASSOCIATED CONDITIONS
- Cold hands: Raynaud's phenomenon
- Dry eyes/mucous membranes: Sjögren's syndrome

PSYCHOSOCIAL IMPACT
- Particularly important in young women
- Confidence, relationships, work
- Depression
- Family planning: infertility/teratogenicity from treatment

SYSTEMIC EFFECTS OF SLE OR TREATMENT
- Renal: hypertension, haematuria, frothy urine/oedema (proteinuria)
- Immunosuppression: skin changes/infections

Examination

FACE
- Malar 'butterfly' rash
- Discoid rash ± scarring (discoid lupus)
- Oral ulceration
- Scarring alopecia

HANDS
- Vasculitic lesions (nail-fold infarcts)
- Jaccoud's arthropathy (mimics rheumatoid arthritis but due to tendon contractures not joint destruction)

SYSTEMIC EFFECTS OF SLE
- Respiratory: percussion and auscultation
  - Pleural effusion
  - Pleural rub
  - Fibrosing alveolitis
- Neurological: finger-nose-finger and/or pronator drift
  - Focal neurology
  - Chorea
  - Ataxia
- Renal:
  - Hypertension

Discussion

DIAGNOSTIC INVESTIGATION
- Serum autoantibodies (ANA and **anti-dsDNA**)

DISEASE ACTIVITY
- Elevated ESR but normal CRP (raised CRP too indicates infection)
- Elevated immunoglobulins

- Reduced complement (C_4)
- U&Es, urine microscopy (glomerulonephritis)

DIAGNOSIS: 4/11 OF AMERICAN COLLEGE OF RHEUMATOLOGY CRITERIA
- Malar rash
- Discoid rash
- Photosensitivity
- Oral ulcers
- Arthritis
- Serositis (pleuritis or pericarditis)
- Renal involvement (proteinuria or cellular casts)
- Neurological disorder (seizures or psychosis)
- Haematological disorder (autoimmune haemolytic anaemia or pancytopenia)
- Immunological disorders (positive anti-dsDNA or anti-Sm antibodies)
- Elevated ANA titre

TREATMENT
- **Mild disease (cutaneous/joint involvement only)**:
  - Topical corticosteroids
  - Hydroxychloroquine
- **Moderate disease (+ other organ involvement)**:
  - Prednisolone
  - Azathioprine
- **Severe disease (+ severe inflammatory involvement of vital organs)**:
  - Methylprednisolone
  - Mycophenolate mofetil (lupus nephritis)
  - Cyclophosphamide
  - Azathioprine

CYCLOPHOSPHAMIDE SIDE EFFECTS
- Haematological and haemorrhagic cystitis
- Infertility
- Teratogenicity

PROGNOSIS
- Good: 90% survival at 10 years

Systemic sclerosis
This woman has painful and swollen hands.

History
HANDS
- Raynaud's **phenomenon** (Raynaud's disease is idiopathic!) Colour change order: white (vasoconstriction) → blue (cyanosis) → red (hyperaemia)
- Ask about function: how does the condition affect ADLs/work, etc.

FUNCTIONAL ENQUIRY
- Hypertension or heart problems
- Lung problems
- Swallowing problems or indigestion

Examination
HANDS
- Sclerodactyly: 'prayer sign'
- Calcinosis (may ulcerate)
- Assess function: holding a cup or pen

FACE
- Tight skin
- Beaked nose
- Microstomia
- Peri-oral furrowing
- Telangiectasia
- Alopecia

OTHER SKIN LESIONS
- Morphoea: focal/generalized patches of sclerotic skin
- En coup de sabre (scar down central forehead)

BLOOD PRESSURE
- Hypertension

RESPIRATORY
- Interstitial fibrosis (fine and bibasal crackles)

CARDIAC
- Pulmonary hypertension (RV heave, loud P_2 and TR)
- Evidence of failure
- Pericarditis (rub)

Discussion
CLASSIFICATION
- **Localized:** morphea to patch of skin only
- **Systemic: limited** and **diffuse**

Limited systemic sclerosis	Diffuse systemic sclerosis
- Distribution limited to below elbows and knees and face	- Widespread cutaneous and early visceral involvement
- Slow progression (years)	- Rapid progression (months)

- Includes **CREST:**
  - **C**alcinosis
  - **R**aynaud's phenomenon
  - **E**sophageal dysmotility
  - **S**clerodactyly
  - **T**elangiectasia

INVESTIGATIONS
- **Autoantibodies:**
  - ANA positive (in 90%)
  - Anti-centromere antibody = limited (in 80%)
  - Scl-70 antibody = diffuse (in 70%)
- **Hand radiographs:** calcinosis
- **Pulmonary disease: lower lobe fibrosis and aspiration pneumonia**:
  - CXR, high-resolution CT scan and pulmonary function tests
- **Gastrointestinal disease: dysmotility and malabsorption**
  - Contrast scans, FBC and B_{12}/folate
- **Renal disease: glomerulonephritis**
  - U&E, urinalysis, urine microscopy (casts) and consider renal biopsy
- **Cardiac disease: myocardial fibrosis and arrhythmias**
  - ECG and echo

TREATMENT
Symptomatic treatment only:

- Camouflage creams
- **Raynaud's therapy:**
  - Gloves, hand-warmers, etc.
  - Calcium-channel blockers
  - ACE-Is
  - Prostacyclin infusion (severe)
- **Renal:**
  - ACE-Is: prevent hypertensive crisis and reduce the mortality from renal failure
- **Gastrointestinal:**
  - Proton-pump inhibitor for oesophageal reflux

PROGNOSIS
Diffuse systemic sclerosis: 50% survival to 5 years (most deaths are due to respiratory failure)

Ankylosing spondylitis
This gentleman complains of back pain.

History
Explore back symptoms

PSYCHOSOCIAL IMPACT
• Work, driving, ADLs, etc.

ASSOCIATED PROBLEMS
• Eye problems: anterior uveitis
• Pneumonia
• Syncope: CHB

Drugs and treatment

Examination
POSTURE
• '?' caused by fixed kyphoscoliosis and loss of lumbar lordosis with extension of cervical spine
• Protuberant abdomen due to diaphragmatic breathing as there is reduced chest expansion (<5 cm increase in girth)
• Increased occiput–wall distance (>5 cm)
• Reduced range of movement throughout entire spine
• **Schöber's test**: Two points marked 15 cm apart on the dorsal spine expand by less than 5 cm on maximum forward flexion

COMPLICATIONS
• **A**nterior uveitis (commonest 30%)
• **A**pical lung fibrosis
• **A**ortic regurgitation (4%): midline sternotomy
• **A**trio-ventricular nodal heart block (10%): pacemaker
• **A**rthritis (may be psoriatic arthropathy)

Discussion
GENETICS
• 90% association with HLA B27

TREATMENT
• Physiotherapy
• Analgesia
• Anti-TNF

Marfan's syndrome
This tall gentleman has a murmur.

History
Family history

FUNCTIONAL ENQUIRY
- Requirement for spectacles or eye surgery
- Cardiac screening with echo or CT surveillance and surgery

Examination
GENERAL (SPOT DIAGNOSIS)
- **Tall** with **long extremities** (arm span > height)

HANDS
- **Arachnodactyly:** can encircle their wrist with thumb and little finger
- **Hyperextensible joints:** thumb able to touch ipsilateral wrist and adduct over the palm with its tip visible at the ulnar boarder

FACE
- **High arched palate** with crowded teeth
- Iridodonesis (with upward lens dislocation)

RESPIRATORY
- Pectus carinatum ('pigeon') or excavatum
- Scoliosis
- Scars from cardiac surgery or chest drains (pneumothorax)

CARDIAC
- Aortic incompetence: collapsing pulse
- Mitral valve prolapse
- Coarctation

ABDOMINAL
- Inguinal herniae and scars

CNS
- Normal IQ

Discussion
GENETICS
- Autosomal dominant and chromosome 15
- Defect in fibrillin protein (connective tissue)

MANAGEMENT
- **Surveillance:** monitoring of aortic root size with annual transthoracic echo
- **Treatment:** β-blockers and angiotensin receptor blocker to slow aortic root dilatation and pre-emptive aortic root surgery to prevent dissection and aortic rupture
- **Screen family members**

DIFFERENTIAL DIAGNOSIS
- Homocystinuria
  - Mental retardation and downward lens dislocation

Paget's disease
This gentleman has had numbness in his fingers.

History
SYMPTOMS
- Usually asymptomatic
- Bone pain and tenderness (2%)

ASSOCIATED CONDITIONS
- Entrapment neuropathy: carpal tunnel syndrome, visual problems, deafness
- CCF: breathlessness

Examination
- Bony enlargement: skull and long bones (sabre tibia)
- Deafness (conductive): hearing-aid
- Pathological fractures: scars

CARDIAC
- High-output heart failure: elevated JVP, SOA, shortness of breath

NEURO
- Entrapment neuropathies: carpal tunnel syndrome

FUNDI
- Optic atrophy and angioid streaks

Discussion
INVESTIGATIONS
- Grossly elevated alkaline phosphatase, normal calcium/phosphate
- Radiology:
  - 'Moth-eaten' on plain films: osteoporosis circumscripta
  - Increase uptake on bone scan

TREATMENT
- Symptomatic: analgesia and hearing-aid
- Bisphosphonates

OTHER COMPLICATIONS
- Osteogenic sarcoma (1%)
- Basilar invagination (cord compression)
- Kidney stones

CAUSES OF SABRE TIBIA
- **Paget's**
- Osteomalacia
- Syphilis

CAUSES OF ANGIOID STREAKS
- **Paget's**
- Pseudoxanthoma elasticum
- Ehlers–Danlos

Other joint problems
This man has problems with his hands.

Tophaceous gout
HISTORY
Cause
- Diet and alcohol: xanthine-rich foods (meat/seafood)
- Drugs: diuretics
- Other conditions: CRF

EXAMINATION
- Asymmetrical swelling of the small joints of the hands and feet (commonly first MTPJ)
- Gouty tophi (chalky white deposits) seen around the joints, ear and tendons
- Reduced movement and function

Associations:
- Obesity
- Hypertension
- Urate stones/nephropathy: nephrectomy scars
- Chronic renal failure: fistulae
- Lymphoproliferative disorders: lymphadenopathy

DISCUSSION
Cause
- Urate excess

Investigation
- Uric acid levels (diagnostically unreliable)
- Synovial fluid: needle-shaped, negatively birefringent crystals
- Radiograph features: 'punched out' periarticular changes

Treatment
- **Acute attack**:
  - Treat the cause
  - Increase hydration
  - High-dose NSAIDs
  - Colchicine and high fluid intake
- **Prevention**:
  - Avoid precipitants
  - Allopurinol (xanthine oxidase inhibitor)

Osteoarthritis
HISTORY
Symptoms
- Stiff, weakness (disuse)
- Not usually painful, red or swollen

Function and social aspects
- Assess function, ask about ADLs and work
- Mobility: walking stick, motorized wheelchair, etc.

Treatments
- Joint replacements
- NSAIDs: side-effects: stomach ulcers, fluid retention, hypertension

EXAMINATION

- Asymmetrical distal interphalangeal joint deformity with Heberden's nodes (and sometimes Bouchard's nodes at the proximal interphalangeal joint)
- Disuse atrophy of hand muscles
- Crepitation, reduced movement and function
- Carpal tunnel syndrome or scars
- Other joint involvement and joint-replacement scars

DISCUSSION

Prevalence: 20% (common)

Radiographic features

- Loss of joint space
- Osteophytes
- Peri-articular sclerosis and cysts

Treatment

- Simple analgesia
- Weight reduction (if OA affects weight-bearing joint)
- Physiotherapy and occupational therapy
- Joint replacement

Diabetic retinopathy

This patient complains of difficulty with their vision.

History

- Ask the patient to detail their problem: duration and nature of visual disturbance
- Establish any underlying medical diagnoses: especially presence or absence of diabetes
- Previous eye problems or treatment
- If they are diabetic: do they have regular retinal screening?

Examination

- Look around for clues: a white stick, braille book or glucometer
- Fundoscopy: check for red reflex (absent if cataract or vitreous haemorrhage)
  Tip: find the disc (inferonasally) then follow each of the four main vessels out to the periphery of the quadrants and finish by examining the macular 'look at the light'
- Check for coexisting hypertensive changes (they always ask!)

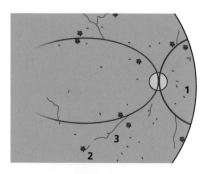

Background retinopathy

1 Hard exudates

2 Blot haemorrhages

3 Microaneurysms

Routine referral to eye clinic.

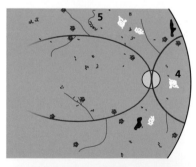

Pre-proliferative retinopathy

Background changes plus

4 Cotton wool spots

5 Flame haemorrhages

Also venous beading and loops and IRMAs (intraretinal microvascular abnormalities).

Urgent referral to ophthalmology.

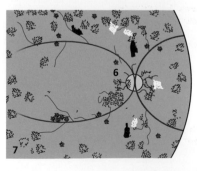

Proliferative retinopathy

Pre-proliferative changes plus

6 Neovascularization of the disc (NVD) and elsewhere

7 Panretinal photocoagulation scars (treatment)

Urgent referral to ophthalmology.

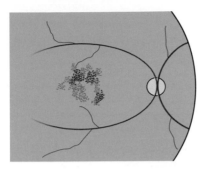

Diabetic maculopathy

Macular oedema or hard exudates within one disc space of the fovea.

Treated with focal photocoagulation.

Urgent referral to ophthalmology.

Discussion
SCREENING
- Annual retinal screening for all patients with diabetes (using retinal photography). Refer to ophthalmology if pre-proliferative retinopathy or changes near the macula
- Background retinopathy usually occurs 10–20 years after diabetes is diagnosed
- Young people with type I diabetes often get proliferative retinopathy whereas older patients with type II diabetes tend to get exudative maculopathy

TREATMENT
Tight glycaemic control
- Improved glycaemic control is associated with less retinopathy
- There may be a transient worsening of the retinopathy initially

Treat other risk factors
- Hypertension; hypercholesterolaemia; smoking cessation
- Accelerated deterioration occurs in poor diabetic control, hypertension and pregnancy

PHOTOCOAGULATION INDICATIONS
- Maculopathy
- Proliferative and pre-proliferative diabetic retinopathy
    Pan-retinal photocoagulation prevents the ischaemic retinal cells secreting angiogenesis factors causing neovascularization. Focal photocoagulation targets problem vessels at risk of bleeding.

COMPLICATIONS OF PROLIFERATIVE DIABETIC RETINOPATHY
- Vitreous haemorrhage (may require vitrectomy)
- Traction retinal detachment
- Neovascular glaucoma due to rubeosis iridis

Cataracts
CLINICAL SIGNS
- Loss of the red reflex
- Cloudy lens
- May have relative afferent pupillary defect (with normal fundi if visible)
- Associations: dystrophia myotonica (bilateral ptosis)

CAUSES
- Congenital (pre-senile): rubella, Turner's syndrome
- Acquired: **age** (usually bilateral), diabetes, drugs (steroids), radiation exposure, trauma and storage disorders

TREATMENT
- Surgery (outpatient):
  - Phacoemulsification with prosthetic lense implantation
  - Yttrium aluminium garnet (YAG) laser capsulotomy

Hyperthyroidism and Graves' disease
This lady has noticed her eyes look different and her neck is swollen.

History
GOITRE
- Usually non-tender (tender = thyroiditis)

EYE PROBLEMS
- See below

THYROID STATUS
- Graves' disease patients may be hyperthyroid, euthyroid or hypothyroid depending on their stage of treatment
- Enquire about: sleep and energy levels, heat intolerance and sweating, agitation, stress and tremor, appetite and weight loss and palpitations

Examination
- Smooth, diffuse goitre

	Specific to Graves'	Hyperthyroidism
Eye signs	Proptosis	Lid retraction
	Chemosis	Lid lag
	Exposure keratitis	
	Ophthalmoplegia	
Peripheral signs	Thyroid acropachy	Agitation
	Pretibial myxoedema	Sweating
		Tremor
		Palmar erythema
		Sinus tachycardia/AF
		Brisk reflexes

EYES
- Keratitis due to poor eye closure
- Optic nerve compression: loss of colour vision initially then development of a central scotoma and reduced visual acuity
- Papilloedema may occur

Discussion
INVESTIGATION
- Thyroid function tests: TSH and T_3/T_4
- Thyroid autoantibodies
- Radioisotope scanning: increased uptake of I^{131} in Graves' disease, reduced in thyroiditis

TREATMENT

- β-Blocker, e.g. propranolol
- Carbimazole or propylthiouracil (both thionamides)
  - **Block and replace** with thyroxine
  - **Titrate** dose and monitor endogenous thyroxine
    Stop at 18 months and assess for return of thyrotoxicosis. One-third of patients will remain euthyroid
  If thyrotoxicosis returns, the options are
  - A repeat course of a thionamide
  - Radioiodine (I^{131}): hypothyroidism common
  - Subtotal thyroidectomy

Severe ophthalmopathy may require high-dose steroids, orbital irradiation or surgical decompression to prevent visual loss

The **NOSPECS** mnemonic for the progression of eye signs in Graves' disease:

No signs or symptoms
Only lid lag/retraction
Soft tissue involvement
Proptosis
Extraocular muscle involvement
Chemosis
Sight loss due to optic nerve compression and atrophy

Hypothyroidism
This patient has been complaining of the cold and has no energy.

History
SYMPTOMS
- Tired and low energy levels
- Cold intolerance
- Weight gain

DRUG HISTORY
- Amiodarone, lithium and anti-thyroid drugs

ASSOCIATED ILLNESSES
- Previously treated thyroid disease
- Autoimmune: Addison's disease, vitiligo and type I diabetes mellitus
- Hypercholesterolaemia
- History of ischaemic heart disease: treatment with thyroxine may precipitate angina

Examination
- **Hands:**
  - Slow pulse
  - Dry skin
  - Cool peripheries
- **Head/face/neck:**
  - 'Peaches and cream' complexion (anaemia and carotenaemia)
  - Eyes: peri-orbital oedema, loss of eyebrows and xanthelasma
  - Thinning hair
  - Goitre or thyroidectomy scar
- **Legs:**
  - Slow relaxing ankle jerk (tested with patient kneeling on a chair)

COMPLICATIONS
- **Cardiac:** pericardial effusion (rub), congestive cardiac failure (oedema)
- **Neurological:** carpel tunnel syndrome (Phalen's/Tinel's test), proximal myopathy (stand from sitting) and ataxia

Discussion
INVESTIGATION
- **Blood:** TSH ($\uparrow$ in thyroid failure, $\downarrow$ in pituitary failure), $T_4 \downarrow$, autoantibodies
  Associations: hyponatraemia, hypercholesterolaemia, macrocytic anaemia, consider short Synacthen test (exclude Addison's)
- **ECG:** pericardial effusion and ischaemia
- **CXR:** pericardial effusion and CCF

MANAGEMENT
- Thyroxine titrated to TSH suppression and clinical response
  NB.   1. Can precipitate angina
        2. Can unmask Addison's disease → crisis

CAUSES
- **Autoimmune:** Hashimoto's thyroiditis (+ goitre) and atrophic hypothyroidism
- **Iatrogenic:** Post-thyroidectomy or I^{131}, amiodarone, lithium and anti-thyroid drugs
- **Iodine deficiency:** dietary ('Derbyshire neck')
- **Dyshormonogenesis**
- **Genetic:** Pendred's syndrome (with deafness)

Acromegaly
This man has been complaining of headaches.*

History
HEADACHE
- Pituitary space-occupying lesion: early morning headache, nausea
- Visual problems: tunnel vision (noticeable when driving)
- Loss of libido and/or lactation

GENERAL OBSERVATIONS
- Change in appearance: photographs
- Tight-fitting jewellery

ASSOCIATED CONDITIONS
- Diabetes mellitus

Examination: 'spot diagnosis'
- **Hands:** large 'spade like', **tight rings***, coarse skin and **sweaty***
- **Face:** prominent supra-orbital ridges, prognathism, widely spaced teeth and macroglossia

COMPLICATIONS TO LOOK FOR: A, B, C ...
Acanthosis nigricans
BP ↑*
Carpal tunnel syndrome
Diabetes mellitus*
Enlarged organs
Field defect*: bitemporal hemianopia
Goitre, **g**astrointestinal malignancy
Heart failure, **h**irsute, **h**ypopituitary
IGF-1 ↑
Joint arthropathy
Kyphosis
Lactation (galactorrhoea)
Myopathy (proximal)

(*Signs of active disease)

Discussion
INVESTIGATIONS
Diagnostic
- **Non-suppression of GH** after an oral glucose tolerance test
- Raised plasma **IGF-1**
- **CT/MRI pituitary fossa:** pituitary adenoma
- Also assess other pituitary functions

Complications
- **CXR:** cardiomegaly
- **ECG:** ischaemia (DM and hypertension)
- **Pituitary function tests:** T_4, ACTH, PRL and testosterone
- **Glucose:** DM
- **Visual perimetry:** bitemporal hemianopia
- **Obstructive sleep apnoea** (in 50%): due to macroglossia

Management
Aim is to normalize GH and IGF-1 levels

1. **Surgery:** trans-sphenoidal approach
   Medical post-op complications:
   - Meningitis
   - Diabetes insipidus
   - Panhypopituitarism
2. **Medical therapy:** somatostatin analogues (Octreotide), dopamine agonists (Cabergoline) and growth hormone receptor antagonists (Pegvisomant)
3. **Radiotherapy** in non-surgical candidates

FOLLOW-UP
Annual GH, PRL, ECG, visual fields and CXR ± CT head

MEN (MULTIPLE ENDOCRINE NEOPLASIA) I
Inherited tumours: autosomal dominant, chromosome 11
- **P**arathyroid hyperplasia (Ca^{2+} ↑)
- **P**ituitary tumours
- **P**ancreatic tumours (gastrinomas)

CAUSES OF MACROGLOSSIA
- **Acromegaly**
- Amyloidosis
- Hypothyroidism
- Down's syndrome

ACANTHOSIS NIGRICANS
- Brown 'velvet-like' skin change found commonly in the axillae.
  Associations:
  - Obesity
  - Type II diabetes mellitus
  - **Acromegaly**
  - Cushing's syndrome
  - Ethnicity: Indian subcontinent
  - Malignancy, e.g. gastric carcinoma and lymphoma

Cushing's disease
This female patient has been gaining weight and has noticed difficulty in getting out of a chair.

History
SYMPTOMS
- Difficulty rising from seated position (proximal myopathy)

DRUG HISTORY
- Exogenous vs endogenous steroid

ASSOCIATED PROBLEMS
- Visual problems: bitemporal hemianopia
- Skin hyperpigmentation
- Diabetes mellitus

DIFFERENTIAL DIAGNOSIS
- Ethanol excess: pseudo-Cushing's

Examination
SPOT DIAGNOSIS
- **Face:** moon-shaped, hirsute, with acne
- **Skin:** bruised, thin, with purple striae
- **Back:** 'buffalo hump'
- **Abdomen:** centripetal obesity
- **Legs:** wasting ('lemon on sticks' body shape) and oedema

COMPLICATIONS
- **Hypertension** (BP)
- **Diabetes mellitus** (random blood glucose)
- **Osteoporosis** (kyphosis)
- **Cellulitis**
- **Proximal myopathy** (stand from sitting)

CAUSE
- **Exogenous:** signs of chronic condition (e.g. RA, COPD) requiring steroids
- **Endogenous:** bitemporal hemianopia and hyperpigmentation (if ACTH ↑)

Discussion
Cushing's disease: glucocorticoid excess due to ACTH secreting pituitary adenoma
Cushing's syndrome: the physical signs of glucocorticoid excess

INVESTIGATION
1. **Confirm high cortisol**
   - 24-hour urinary collection
   - Low dose (for 48 hours) or overnight dexamethasone suppression test
   Suppressed cortisol: alcohol/depression/obesity ('pseudo-Cushing's')
2. **If elevated cortisol confirmed, then identify cause:**
   - **ACTH level**
     o **High:** ectopic ACTH secreting tumour or pituitary adenoma
     o **Low:** adrenal adenoma/carcinoma
   - **MRI pituitary fossa ± adrenal CT ± whole body CT** to locate lesion
   - **Bilateral inferior petrosal sinus vein sampling** (best test to confirm pituitary vs ectopic origin; may also lateralise pituitary adenoma)
   - **High-dose dexamethasone suppression test may help >50% suppressed cortisol:** Cushing's disease

Treatment
Surgical: Trans-sphenoidal approach to remove pituitary tumours. Adrenalectomy for adrenal tumours
Nelson's syndrome: bilateral adrenalectomy (scars) to treat Cushing's disease, causing massive production of ACTH (and melanocyte-stimulating hormone), due to lack of feedback inhibition, leading to hyper-pigmentation and pituitary overgrowth
Pituitary irradiation
Medical: Metyrapone

PROGNOSIS
Untreated Cushing's syndrome: 50% mortality at 5 years (usually due to accelerated ischaemic heart disease secondary to diabetes and hypertension)

CAUSES OF PROXIMAL MYOPATHY
- **Inherited:**
  - Myotonic dystrophy
  - Muscular dystrophy
- **Endocrine:**
  - **Cushing's syndrome**
  - Hyperparathyroidism
  - Thyrotoxicosis
  - Diabetic amyotrophy
- **Inflammatory:**
  - Polymyositis
  - Rheumatoid arthritis
- **Metabolic:**
  - Osteomalacia
- **Malignancy:**
  - Paraneoplastic
  - Lambert–Eaton myasthenic syndrome
- **Drugs:**
  - Alcohol
  - Steroids

Addison's disease

Examine this man; he was admitted as an emergency 4 days ago with postural hypotension.

History

SYMPTOMS
- Fatigue, muscle weakness, low mood, loss of appetite, weight loss, thirst (dehydration)
- Darkened skin (Addison's disease)
- Fainting or cramps

CAUSE
- Known Addison's disease on steroid
- Other autoimmune disease e.g. hypothyroidism, type I diabetes mellitus and vitiligo
- TB or metastasis

DIFFERENTIAL DIAGNOSIS
- Secondary adrenal insufficiency: pituitary adenoma or sudden discontinuation of steroid

Examination
- Medic alert bracelet
- Hyper-pigmentation: palmar creases, scars, nipples and buccal mucosa
- Postural hypotension
- Visual fields: bitemporal hemianopia (pituitary adenoma)

CAUSE
- Signs of other associated autoimmune diseases
- Signs of TB or malignancy

Discussion

ADDISON'S DISEASE: PRIMARY ADRENAL INSUFFICIENCY
- Pigmentation due to a lack of feedback inhibition by cortisol on the pituitary, leading to raised ACTH and melanocyte-stimulating hormone
- In 80% of cases Addison's disease is due to an autoimmune process. Other causes include adrenal metastases, adrenal tuberculosis, amyloidosis, adrenalectomy and Waterhouse–Friederichsen syndrome (meningococcal sepsis and adrenal infarction)

INVESTIGATION ORDER
- **8 am cortisol:** no morning elevation suggests Addison's disease (unreliable)
- **Short Synacthen® test**
  ○ **Exclude Addison's disease** if cortisol rises to adequate levels
- **Long Synacthen® test**
  ○ **Diagnose Addison's disease** if cortisol does not rise to adequate levels
- **Adrenal imaging (primary) and/or pituitary imaging (secondary) with MRI or CT**

OTHER TESTS
Blood: eosinophilia, ↓ Na$^+$ (kidney loss), ↑ K$^+$, ↑ urea (dehydration), ↓ glucose, adrenal autoantibodies (if autoimmune cause), thyroid function tests (hypothyroidism)
CXR: Malignancy or TB

TREATMENT
Acute (adrenal crisis)
- 0.9% saline IV rehydration +++ and glucose
- Hydrocortisone

- Treatment may unmask diabetes insipidus (cortisol is required to excrete a water load)
- Anti-TB treatment increases the clearance of steroid, therefore higher doses required

Chronic
- **Education:** compliance, increase steroid dose if 'ill', steroid card, medic alert bracelet
- Titrate maintenance hydrocortisone (and fludrocortisone) dose to levels/response

Prognosis
- Normal life expectancy

Sickle cell disease

Examine this 25 year old man who has been admitted with chest and bone pain in association with worsening shortness of breath.

History
- Longstanding fatigue with breathlessness on exertion
- 12-hour history of sudden-onset thigh bone pain and pleuritic chest pain
- Associated with worsening shortness of breath
- Events preceded by a viral prodrome
- History of leg ulcers and priapism

Examination
- Fever
- Dyspnoeic
- Jaundice
- Pale conjunctiva
- Raised JVP, pansystolic murmur loudest at left sternal edge (tricuspid regurgitation)
- Reduced chest expansion due to pain with coarse expiratory crackles
- Small, crusted ulcers on lower third of legs

Differential diagnosis
- Sickle cell disease with a vaso-occlusive sickle crisis
- Acute sickle cell chest crisis
- Sickle cell crisis with a history of pulmonary hypertension
- Acute pulmonary embolism in the context of a vaso-occlusive sickle crisis

Discussion
- Vaso-occlusive crisis occurs as a result of sickling in the small vessels of any organ; lungs, kidney and bone most common
- Often precipitated by a viral illness, exercise or hypoxia
- Leg ulcers are due to ischaemia
- High mortality associated with the development of chest crises in adulthood
- Worse prognosis for patients with triad of leg ulcers, priapism and pulmonary hypertension

INVESTIGATIONS
- Blood tests: low Hb; high WCC and CRP; renal impairment; sickling on blood film
- CXR: linear atelectasis in a chest crisis; cardiomegaly: cardiac size proportional to degree of longstanding anaemia
- Urinalysis: microscopic haematuria if renal involvement in crisis
- Arterial blood gas: type I respiratory failure
- Echocardiogram: dilated right ventricle with impaired systolic function; raised peak tricuspid regurgitant velocity: abnormal range for sickle cell patients is lower than other populations; i.e. >2.7 m/s abnormal
- Computed tomography pulmonary angiography: linear atelectasis with patchy consolidation ± acute pulmonary embolism

TREATMENT
- Oxygen ± continuous positive airways pressure
- Intravenous fluids
- Analgesia
- Antibiotics if evidence of infection
- Blood transfusion/exchange transfusion depending on degree of anaemia and severity of crisis

- Hydroxycarbamide or exchange transfusion programme if frequent crises or other features suggestive of a poor prognosis
- Long-term treatment with folic acid and penicillin as patient will have features of hyposplenism
- May need further investigation of possible pulmonary hypertension if raised peak tricuspid regurgitant velocity, including right heart catheterization, after the acute event

PROGNOSIS
- HbSS ≈40–50 years old
- Worse prognosis with frequent chest crises or following development of pulmonary hypertension

Index

Cases for PACES, Third Edition. Stephen Hoole, Andrew Fry and Rachel Davies.
© 2015 John Wiley & Sons, Ltd. Published 2015 by John Wiley & Sons, Ltd.